O P M L

OXFORD PAIN MANAGEMENT LIBRARY

Cancer-related
Bone Pain

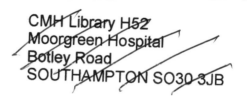
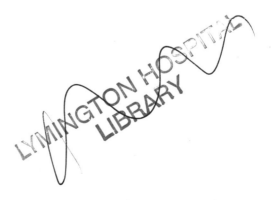

Oxford University Press makes no representation, express or implied, that the drug dosages in this book are correct. Readers must therefore always check the product information and clinical procedures with the most up-to-date published product information and data sheets provided by the manufacturers and the most recent codes of conduct and safety regulations. The authors and the publishers do not accept responsibility or legal liability for any errors in the text or for the misuse or misapplication of material in this work.

▶ Except where otherwise stated, drug doses and recommendations are for the non-pregnant adult who is not breast-feeding.

O P M L

OXFORD PAIN MANAGEMENT LIBRARY

Cancer-related Bone Pain

Editor

Dr Andrew Davies

Consultant in Palliative Medicine,
The Royal Marsden Hospital,
Sutton, UK.

OXFORD
UNIVERSITY PRESS

OXFORD
UNIVERSITY PRESS

Great Clarendon Street, Oxford OX2 6DP

Oxford University Press is a department of the University of Oxford.
It furthers the University's objective of excellence in research, scholarship,
and education by publishing worldwide in

Oxford New York

Auckland Cape Town Dar es Salaam Hong Kong Karachi
Kuala Lumpur Madrid Melbourne Mexico City Nairobi
New Delhi Shanghai Taipei Toronto

With offices in

Argentina Austria Brazil Chile Czech Republic France Greece
Guatemala Hungary Italy Japan Poland Portugal Singapore
South Korea Switzerland Thailand Turkey Ukraine Vietnam

Oxford is a registered trade mark of Oxford University Press
in the UK and in certain other countries

Published in the United States
by Oxford University Press Inc., New York

British Library Cataloguing in Publication Data

Data available

Library of Congress Cataloging in Publication Data

Data available

Typeset by Newgen Imaging Systems (P) Ltd, Chennai, India
Printed in China
on acid-free paper through
Phoenix Offset

ISBN 978-0-19-921573-7

10 9 8 7 6 5 4 3 2 1

Whilst every effort has been made to ensure that the contents of this book are as
complete, accurate and-up-to-date as possible at the date of writing. Oxford
University Press is not able to give any guarantee or assurance that such is the case.
Readers are urged to take appropriately qualified medical advice in all cases. The
information in this book is intended to be useful to the general reader, but should
not be used as a means of self-diagnosis or for the prescription of medication.

Contents

Contributors

Wisam Al-Hakim
Clinical Research Fellow in
Orthopaedic surgery
Royal National Orthopaedic
Hospital, Stanmore, UK
*Chapter 10 Orthopaedic
interventions*

Timothy Briggs
Consultant in Orthopaedic
surgery
Royal National Orthopaedic
Hospital, Stanmore, UK
*Chapter 10 Orthopaedic
interventions*

James Crawshaw
SpR in Radiology
The Royal Marsden Hospital,
Sutton, UK
Chapter 5 Radiology

Andrew Davies
Consultant in Palliative Medicine
The Royal Marsden Hospital,
Sutton, UK
Chapter 1 Introduction
*Chapter 4 General principles of
management*

Marie T. Fallon
Professor of Palliative Medicine
Edinburgh Cancer Centre,
Edinburgh, UK
Chapter 3 Clinical features

Paul Farquhar-Smith
Consultant Anaesthetist
The Royal Marsden Hospital,
Sutton, UK
*Chapter 9 Anaesthetic/
interventional techniques*

Robert Huddart
Consultant in Clinical Oncology
The Royal Marsden Hospital,
Sutton, UK
Chapter 8 Radiotherapy

Jacob Jagiello
Clinical Research Fellow in
Orthopaedic surgery
Royal National Orthopaedic
Hospital, Stanmore, UK
*Chapter 10 Orthopaedic
Interventions*

Sandra McConnell
SpR in Palliative Medicine
Edinburgh Oncology Centre,
Edinburgh, UK
Chapter 3 Clinical features

David MacVicar
Consultant Radiologist
The Royal Marsden Hospital,
Sutton, UK
Chapter 5 Radiology

Catherine E. Urch
Consultant in Palliative
Medicine
St Mary's and Royal Brompton
Hospitals, London, UK
Chapter 2 Pathophysiology

Nicholas Van As
SpR in Clinical Oncology
The Royal Marsden Hospital,
Sutton, UK
Chapter 8 Radiotherapy

Joanna Vriens
SpR in Palliative Medicine
The Royal Marsden Hospital,
Sutton, UK
Chapter 1 Introduction

Rebecca Wong
Associate Professor of
Radiation Oncology
Princess Margaret Hospital,
Toronto, Canada
*Chapter 7 Bisphosphonates for
bone pain*

John Zeppetella
Consultant in Palliative
Medicine
St Clare Hospice,
Hastingwood, UK
*Chapter 6 Conventional
analgesics for bone pain*

Chapter 1

Introduction

Andrew Davies and Joanna Vriens

1.1 Introduction

Over the last few years there has been an increasing interest in the phenomenon of cancer-related bone pain, generated by a better understanding of the pathophysiology of bone pain (Urch, 2004), and fuelled by an increasing number of options for the management of bone pain (e.g. radionuclides, bisphosphonates) (Mercadante, 1997).

The aim of this chapter is to provide an introduction to the skeletal system, and to the problem of cancer-related pain (also known as cancer-induced bone pain or CIBP). Subsequent chapters will discuss in detail the pathophysiology, clinical features, investigation, and management of this particular type of pain.

1.2 Anatomy and physiology

The adult skeleton consists of 206 individual bones, and is sub-divided into the axial skeleton (80 bones), and the appendicular skeleton (126 bones) (Tortora and Derrickson, 2006). The axial skeleton consists of the bones of the skull, the vertebral column, and the thoracic cage, as well as the hyoid bone and the auditory ossicles; the appendicular skeleton consists of the bones of the shoulder girdle, the upper limbs, the pelvic girdle, and the lower limbs (see Figure 1.1). The paediatric skeleton consists of a greater number of individual bones, but many of these will fuse together as the child develops into an adult.

The macroscopic structure of a long bone (i.e. humerus) is shown in Figure 1.2. The body of the bone is called the diaphysis, and the ends of the bone are called the epiphyses; the metaphyses are the regions between the diaphysis and the epiphyses, and in adults they contain the epiphyseal line which represents the mature epiphyseal plate (Tortora and Derrickson, 2006). The connective sheath that surrounds the bone is called the periosteum, and the membrane that lines the medullary cavity (also known as the marrow cavity) is called the endosteum. The bone as a whole has an extensive blood supply, whilst the periosteum has a prominent nerve supply.

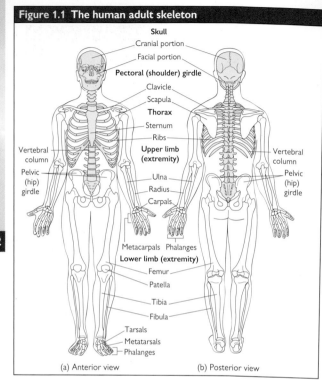

Figure 1.1 The human adult skeleton

Skull
Cranial portion
Facial portion
Pectoral (shoulder) girdle
Clavicle
Scapula
Thorax
Sternum
Ribs
Upper limb (extremity)
Ulna
Radius
Carpals
Metacarpals Phalanges
Lower limb (extremity)
Femur
Patella
Tibia
Fibula
Tarsals
Metatarsals
Phalanges

Vertebral column
Pelvic (hip) girdle

(a) Anterior view   (b) Posterior view

Bone is made up of specialized cells interspersed in extracellular matrix (Tortora and Derrickson, 2006). The specialized cells include: (a) osteogenic cells—these are stem cells that develop into osteoblasts; (b) osteoblasts—these cells are responsible for the synthesis of the extracellular matrix, and they go on to develop into osteocytes; (c) osteocytes—these cells are responsible for maintenance of bone metabolism; (d) osteoclasts—these cells are responsible for the breakdown of the extracellular matrix. The extracellular matrix includes: (a) mineral (e.g. hydroxyapatite), 50%; (b) collagen, 25%; and (c) water, 25%.

Bone is also made up a number of small spaces, which contain the blood vessels and the bone marrow (Tortora and Derrickson, 2006). Compact bone refers to bone that has relatively few of these spaces; it accounts for 80% of the bone, is found particularly in diaphysis of the long bones, and provides much of the strength of the bone.

Figure 1.1 is reproduced from Tortora, G.J., and Derrickson, B. (2006). *Principles of Anatomy and Physiology* 11th edition, ISBN 0471689343, with permission of John Wiley & Sons, Inc.

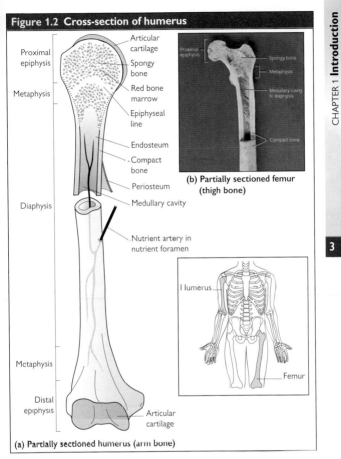

Figure 1.2 Cross-section of humerus

Proximal epiphysis

Metaphysis

Diaphysis

Metaphysis

Distal epiphysis

Articular cartilage
Spongy bone
Red bone marrow
Epiphyseal line
Endosteum
Compact bone
Periosteum
Medullary cavity
Nutrient artery in nutrient foramen
Articular cartilage

(b) Partially sectioned femur (thigh bone)

Humerus

Femur

(a) Partially sectioned humerus (arm bone)

In contrast, spongy bone refers to bone that has more of these spaces; it accounts for 20% of the bone, is found in various areas of the long/other type of bones, and contains the bone marrow (as well as providing some of the strength of the bone).

1.3 Epidemiology and clinical features

Primary malignant tumours of the bone are extremely uncommon (e.g. osteosarcoma, Ewing's sarcoma). For example, only 408 cases of primary malignant tumour of the bone (and of the articular cartilage)

Figure 1.2 is reproduced from Tortora, G.J., and Derrickson, B. (2006). *Principles of Anatomy and Physiology* 11th edition, ISBN 0471689343, with permission of John Wiley & Sons, Inc.

were registered in England during 2003 [Office for National Statistics (ONS), 2005]. Indeed, these tumours represented ~0.14% tumours registered in is dependent on the primary tumour (type, histology), the duration of disease, and also the diagnostic method utilized (e.g. bone scan, England during 2003 (ONS, 2005).

In contrast, secondary (metastatic) tumours of the bone are very common. The bone is the third most common site of metastatic involvement (after the lungs and the liver) (Tubiana-Hulin, 1991). The incidence of bone metastases post mortem examination (Galasko, 1986).

Bone metastases are particularly common in patients with prostate, breast, thyroid, kidney, and lung tumours. For example, studies suggest that between 54–85% of patients with prostate cancer have evidence of bone metastases on post-mortem examination (Tubiana-Hulin, 1991). The corresponding figures for other types of cancer are: breast, 47–85%; thyroid, 28–60%; kidney, 33–40%; lung, 32–40% (Tubiana-Hulin, 1991). Bone pain is also common in patients with myeloma (MacLennan et al., 1994), and may occur in patients with other haematological malignancies (Jean-Baptiste and De Ceulaer, 2000).

Bone metastases are commoner in axial skeleton than in appendicular skeleton, although they may occur in any bone (Galasko, 1986). Table 1.1 shows the distribution of skeletal metastases in a post-mortem study of patients with various types of cancer (Willis, 1973). In most series, the vertebral column is the most common site of bone metastases, and the most common local site of involvement is the lumbar vertebrae, then the thoracic vertebrae, then the cervical vertebrae, and then the sacrum (Galasko, 1986).

Bone pain is the most common type of pain in patients with cancer (Foley, 2004). However, not all bone tumours are associated with bone pain. For example, one study of breast cancer patients found that only 68% patients with a positive bone scan were experiencing bone pain (Front et al., 1979). Moreover, only 32% lesions on the bone scans were associated with bone pain (Front et al., 1979).

Patients with bone pain may experience a constant background pain as well as intermittent 'breakthrough pain'. Indeed, movement-related breakthrough pain ('volitional incident pain') is a major cause of morbidity, particularly as this type of pain can be very difficult to control (Davies, 2006). The clinical features of bone pain are discussed in more detail in Chapter 3.

Table 1.1 Distribution of bone metastases at post-mortem in cancer patients with metastatic bone disease (Willis, 1973)

Anatomical site	Metastases present (n = 68)
Vertebrae*	42 (62%)
Ribs	39 (57%)
Skull	24 (35%)
Femur	15 (22%)
Pelvis	13 (19%)
Humerus	7 (10%)
Sternum	7 (10%)
Clavicle	4 (6%)
Scapula	2 (3%)

* Lumbar vertebrae, 36; thoracic vertebrae, 25; cervical vertebrae, 15; sacrum, 4.

References

Davies, A.N. (2006). Introduction. In: Davies, A.N. (ed.) *Cancer-related breakthrough pain*, pp. 1–11. Oxford University Press, Oxford.

Foley, K.M. (2004). Acute and chronic cancer pain syndromes. In: Doyle, D., Hanks, G., Cherny, N., and Calman, K. (ed.) *Oxford Textbook of Palliative Medicine* (3rd edn), pp. 298–316. Oxford University Press, Oxford.

Front, D., Schneck, S.O., Frankel A., and Robinson, E. (1979). Bone metastases and bone pain in breast cancer. *JAMA*, **242**, 1747–8.

Galasko, C.A. (1986). *Skeletal metastases*. Butterworths, London.

Jean-Baptiste, G. and De Ceulaer K (2000). Osteoarticular disorders of haematological origin. Best Pract. Res. Clin. Rheumatol., **14**, 307 23.

MacLennan, I.C., Drayson, M., and Dunn, J. (1994). Multiple myeloma. *DMJ*, **300**, 1033–6.

Mercadante S (1997). Malignant bone pain: pathophysiology and treatment. *Pain*, **69**, 1–18.

Office for National Statistics (2005). *Cancer statistics: registrations*. Office for National Statistics, London.

Tortora, G.J., and Derrickson, B. (2006). Principles of Anatomy and Physiology. Wiley, Hoboken.

Tubiana-Hulin, M. (1991). Incidence, prevalence and distribution of bone metastases. *Bone*, **12** (Suppl. 1), S9–10.

Urch, C. (2004). The pathophysiology of cancer-induced bone pain: current understanding. *Palliat. Med.*, **18**, 267–74.

Willis, R.A. (1973). *The spread of tumours in the human body* (3rd edn). Butterworths, London.

Chapter 2

Pathophysiology

Catherine E. Urch

2.1 Introduction

The development of suitable animal models of cancer-induced bone pain (CIBP) has led to an unprecedented increase in our understanding of the pathophysiology of this type of pain. The results of animal studies suggest that CIBP is a unique and complex pain state, with features of both inflammatory and neuropathic pain; they also suggest the possibility of novel therapeutics to treat this type of pain. This chapter will give a brief overview of the current understanding of the pathophysiology of CIBP.

2.2 Animal models of CIBP

As discussed above, animal models have allowed insight into the unique pathophysiology of CIBP. Schwei et al. (1999) reported a method of local infusion of cancer (osteosarcoma) cells into a single bone of a mouse: they demonstrated that this method resulted in a systemically well animal, and localized bone pain, which provided for the first time a suitable model to investigate the pathophysiology of CIBP. In this early model the bone was not plugged, and a local escape of tumour was noted (but not distant metastases).

The osteosarcoma cells were infused directly into the medulla of a mouse femur, and from day 14 onwards the animals demonstrated increasing severe pain behaviours (that correlated with the degree of bone destruction). These were quantified according to limp on walking, flinching or vocalization on palpation, withdrawal threshold to punctate mechanical pressure (von Frey filaments), and spontaneous licking and flinching. These pain behaviours are taken as correlates of human movement-induced pain, point tenderness, tonic (background) pain, and spontaneous pain respectively.

Since 1999 several models using the same principle of local infusion have been described, although the bone is now uniformly plugged after infusion. Models include rat breast carcinoma (MRMT-1 cell line) injected into the tibia of rats, and fibrosarcoma, melanoma, and prostate carcinoma injected into the humerus or femur of mice (Medhurst et al., 2002; Sabino et al., 2003; Sevcik et al., 2005). In all these models the clinical situation parallels the bone destruction leading to pathological fracture.

One main difference between these animal models and the clinical situation in man is the lack of non-painful metastases, which is a common finding in man, and which could reveal much about the inhibitory controls governing CIBP.

2.3 Peripheral mechanisms

It has been recently established that the periosteum and the mineralized bone are richly innervated by primary afferent fibres (Aδ, C, sympathetic fibres). Whilst the periosteum is the most densely innovated, the bone marrow contains the greatest number (when volume is considered) followed by the mineralized bone (Mach et al., 2002). The primary afferents transmit noxious stimuli, activated at specific thresholds, and coded for intensity and duration of stimuli.

The Aδ fibres are fully functional, expressing amongst others neuropeptide Y and vasoactive intestinal peptide (VIP) neurotransmitters (Hohmann et al., 1986; Bjurholm et al., 1988; Hukkanen et al., 1992). Only peptidergic C fibres appear to be present, expressing calcitonin gene-related peptide (CGRP); no IB4-positive C fibres appear to be present (Hill and Elde, 1991). The neuronal activation and release of VIP, CGRP and substance P into bones appears to be vital for embryological development, post-natal development and bone metabolism (Chenu et al., 1998; Serre et al., 1999).

Tumours growing within the medullary space of the bone, actively alter the melieu, interact with the normal osteoclast/osteoblast balance, and directly and indirectly activate the nociceptive primary afferents (Figure 2.1).

Tumour cells have been shown to release a host of growth factors (e.g. nerve-growth factor, granulocyte-colony stimulating factor), cytokines (e.g. tumour necrosis factor: TNF), interleukins (e.g. IL-1, IL-6), prostanoids, and endothelins (Suzuki and Yamada, 1994; Mantyh et al., 2002). Many of these are important in maintaining tumour growth and migration, but they also directly interact with the primary afferents triggering depolarization and transmission.

Prostanoids are pro-inflammatory derivatives of arachidonic acid, which are formed by the action of cyclo-oxygenase. They have been shown to activate prostanoid receptors on primary afferents and induce pain behaviours (Murata et al., 1997; Bley et al., 1998). Endothelins are vital to tumour growth and invasion (Asham et al., 1998). They promote pain behaviours via activation of the endothelin receptors on primary afferents (Davar et al., 1998; De-Melo et al., 1998). Human prostate carcinoma has been shown to express high levels of endothelins, and the plasma level of endothelin correlates with the severity of pain (Nelson et al., 1995; Lassiter and Carducci, 2003).

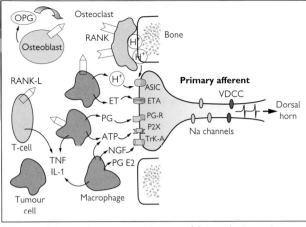

Figure 2.1 Schematic diagram summarizing some of the complex interactions between the invading tumour cells, the recruited immune response, the activated osteoclasts/osteoblasts and the primary afferent nerve fibres.

Key: TNF = tumor necrosis factor IL-1 = interleukin 1 OPG = osteoprotegerin RANK = recetor activator for nuclear factor KB RANK-L = RANK ligand H^+ = proton ASIC = acid-sensing ion channel ET = endothlins ETA = endothelin receptor ATP = adenosine triphoshate NGF = nerve growth factor receptor NA = sodium VDCC = voltage dependent calcium channel

In addition the tumour cells release protons, which reduce the surrounding pH to ≤5 (Griffiths, 1991). This will directly activate primary afferents via the acid-sensing ion channels, and also allow activation of osteoclasts and direct resorption of bone (Reeh and Steen, 1996; Olson et al., 1998; Takayanagi, 2005). As tumour cells outgrow the nutrient supply, cell death occurs with release of the contents of the cells, including adenosine triphosphate, which is another potent activator of primary afferents via the P_2X receptor (North, 2002; Gallagher, 2004).

Invading tumours also elicit a vigorous immune response, albeit ineffective at obliterating the cancer. The invasion of active T cells, macrophages and natural killer cells, adds an inflammatory dimension to the primary afferent activation and interaction (Ogmundsdottir, 2001). For example, cytokines are released by inflammatory cells (e.g. TNF). TNF will enhance the immune response, lead to release of other cytokines, chemokines, and interleukins, and have an effect on primary afferents leading to activation (Mocellin et al., 2005).

The normal architecture of bone is maintained/renewed through activation of osteoclasts (involved in bone resorption) and osteoblasts (involved in new bone formation) (Szczesny, 2002). Any microfracture, or alteration in weight load, leads to the migration and activation of the osteoclasts. Osteoclast activation, and growth factor release (secondary to bone resorption), activates osteoblasts, which secrete osteoid matrix. Over time this is mineralized to form new bone. The balance is strictly maintained with numerous positive and negative feedback loops (Troen, 2003). It should be noted that systemic influences such as hormones (parathyroid hormone, calcitonin, oestrogen, steroids), vitamins (vitamin D), and immobility amongst others also impact on the resorption or formation of bones.

One of the main pathways for achieving balanced osteoclast–osteoblast activation is via the RANK–RANK L system. RANK refers to the receptor activator for nuclear factor κB, which is expressed on precursor and mature osteoclasts; RANK L refers to the RANK ligand (also known as osteoprotegerin ligand or OPGL), which is found on osteoblasts and activated T cells (Honore et al., 2000a; Thompson and Tonge, 2000). Osteoclast formation and activation requires macrophage colony stimulating factor, and the interaction between the RANK and RANK-L, and an acid environment (pH <6) (Lacey et al., 1998; Yasuda et al., 1998).

A balance is maintained by the cytokine osteoprotegerin (OPG), which binds and sequesters RANK-L, thus preventing further RANK activation. OPG is normally released by active osteoblasts (Thompson and Tonge, 2000). Many tumours engage in activation of osteoclasts, and disturbance of the normal osteoblast–osteoclast balance, via secretion of RANK-L; tumours also recruit activated T cells into the tumour area, which also express RANK-L (Standal et al., 2002; Sezer et al., 2003). Interestingly, it was reported that injection of exogenous OPG reduced the pain behaviour in mice injected with osteosarcoma cells (Honore et al., 2000a). In addition, clinical trials confirm the role of OPG in myeloma, with reported reduction in bone pain with treatment (Body et al., 2003; Sezer et al., 2003).

As the tumour continues to grow, and osteoclasts continue to destroy bone, primary afferents will be destroyed. The tumour may compress, invade, or cause ischaemia or proteolysis of the nerve fibres. This will cause direct activation of the primary afferents (i.e. 'neuropathic' pain) (Mantyh, 2002). The primary afferents are dynamic or 'plastic', and alter their phenotype in response to sustained injury. Thus neurons may become more responsive to lower thresholds, but also silent (or sleeping) nociceptors may become activated (Schmidt et al., 2000). This, together with central changes, produces the effect of primary and secondary peripheral hyperalgesia, characterized by reduced thresholds (to mechanical, thermal and dynamic stimuli), increased receptive field size, and increased area of sensitivity (Herrero et al., 2000).

2.4 **Dorsal horn mechanisms**

Information from animal models suggests that the dorsal horn of the spinal cord also undergoes significant alterations, which renders it hyperexcitable. Thus, spinal cord neurons that would normally only be responsive to noxious stimuli become responsive to non-noxious stimuli. Results in the mouse osteosarcoma model indicate that the alterations in the dorsal horn are different from that seen in inflammatory and neuropathy pain (Honore et al., 2000c): up-regulation of dynorphin, a pro-hyperalgesic peptide, is observed in CIBP, inflammatory and neuropathy pain (Honore et al., 2000b); however, pro-inflammatory changes such as up-regulation of CGRP, or pro-neuropathic changes such as increased neuropeptide Y, are not seen in CIBP (Honore et al., 2000c; Luger et al., 2001). Evidence for central sensitization (alterations within the dorsal horn leading to a pro-excitatory state) is found in the increased expression of c fos, and the internalization of the substance P–neurokinin 1 receptor complex after noxious stimuli (Honore and Mantyh, 2000).

In addition, in vivo electrophysiology of individual dorsal horn neurons has indicated a profound change with increased excitation within lamina I and V (Urch et al., 2003). Lamina I neurons exhibited a greater alteration, which has not been reported in either inflammation or neuropathy. Lamina I neurons can be divided into those that respond to only noxious stimuli (nociceptive specific: NS), or those that respond to both innocuous and noxious stimuli (wide-dynamic range: WDR). In the normal dorsal horn the ratio of NS:WDR is 75%:25%. However, in the rat breast cancer model of CIBP, the ratio alters to 53%:47% (NS:WDR). In addition, the WDR neurons show an increased response to electrical and mechanical stimuli (Urch et al., 2003). This alteration in lamina I responses has been shown to parallel the development of hyperalgesia and allodynia [Donovan-Rodriguez et al., 2004].

Spinal astrocyte activation has also been demonstrated in the murine osteosarcoma model (Honore et al., 2000c). Glia, both astrocytes and microglia, in the spinal cord have been shown to be involved in the development of persistent pain in tissue inflammation and nerve injury (Watkins et al., 2001). In a prostate cancer model in rats, both glial fibrillary acidic protein (an astrocyte marker) and OX-42 (a microglial marker) were enhanced on the ipsilateral but not contralateral side, and the glia were actively secreting the pro-excitatory IL-1β (Zhang et al., 2005). Further work is needed to explore the role of glia in the generation and maintenance of hyperalgesia in CIBP, and also the use of antagonists of glial activation for the treatment of CIBP (Sweitzer et al., 2001; Ledeboer et al., 2005).

2.5 **Central mechanisms**

The pathophysiological alterations in CIBP are not merely confined to the periphery, but extend to the brain and back via alteration in the descending facilitation and inhibition pathways (Apkarian et al., 2005). The ascending pathway from lamina I projecting neurons is predominantly to the parabrachial area (e.g. hypothalamus, amygdala), which accounts for the affective component of pain experience (Gauriau and Bernard, 2002): this may account for the perception of CIBP as disturbing and unpleasant, with increased alterations in affect, anxiety and depression (Portenoy and Hagen, 1990). The higher centre alterations in CIBP have yet to be explored thoroughly.

References

Apkarian, A.V., Bushnell, M.C., Treede, R.D., and Zubieta, J.K. (2005). Human brain mechanisms of pain perception and regulation in health and disease. *Eur. J. Pain*, **9**, 463–84.

Asham, E.H., Loizidou, M., and Taylor, I. (1998). Endothelin-1 and tumour development. *Eur. J. Surg. Oncol.*, **24**, 57–60.

Bjurholm, A., Kreicbergs, A., Terenius, L., Goldstein, M., and Schultzberg, M. (1988). Neuropeptide Y-, tyrosine hydroxylase- and vasoactive intestinal polypeptide-immunoreactive nerves in bone and surrounding tissues. *J. Autonom. Nerv. Syst.*, **25**, 119–25.

Bley, K.R., Hunter, J.C., Eglen, R.M., and Smith, J.A. (1998). The role of IP prostanoid receptors in inflammatory pain. *Trends Pharmacol. Sci.*, **19**, 141–7.

Body, J.J., Greipp, P., Coleman, R.E. et al. (2003). A phase I study of AMGN-0007, a recombinant osteoprotegerin construct, in patients with multiple myeloma or breast carcinoma related bone metastases. *Cancer*, **97** (3 Suppl.), 887–92.

Chenu, C., Serre, C.M., Raynal, C., Burt-Pichat, B., and Delmas, P.D. (1998). Glutamate receptors are expressed by bone cells and are involved in bone resorption. *Bone*, **22**, 295–9.

Davar, G., Hans, G., Fareed, M.U., Sinnott, C., and Strichartz, G. (1998). Behavioral signs of acute pain produced by application of endothelin-1 to rat sciatic nerve. *Neuroreport*, **9**, 2279–83.

De-Melo, J.D., Tonussi, C.R., D'Orleans-Juste, P., and Rae, G.A. (1998). Articular nociception induced by endothelin-1, carrageenan and LPS in naive and previously inflamed knee-joints in the rat: inhibition by endothelin receptor antagonists. *Pain*, **77**, 261–9.

Donovan-Rodriguez, T., Dickenson, A.H., and Urch, C.E. (2004). Superficial dorsal horn neuronal responses and the emergence of behavioural hyperalgesia in a rat model of cancer-induced bone pain. *Neurosci. Lett.*, **360**, 29–32.

Gallagher, J.A. (2004). ATP P2 receptors and regulation of bone effector cells. *J. Musculoskel Neuronal Interact.*, **4**, 125–7.

Gauriau, C., and Bernard, J.F. (2002). Pain pathways and parabrachial circuits in the rat. *Exp. Physiol.*, **87**, 251–8.

Griffiths, J.R. (1991). Are cancer cells acidic? *Br. J. Cancer*, **64**, 425–7.

Herrero, J.F., Laird, J.M., and Lopez-Garcia J.A. (2000). Wind-up of spinal cord neurones and pain sensation: much ado about something? *Progr. Neurobiol.*, **61**, 169–203.

Hill, E.L. and Elde, R. (1991). Distribution of CGRP-, VIP-, D beta H-, SP-, and NPY- immunoreactive nerves in the periosteum of the rat. *Cell Tiss Res.*, **264**, 469–80.

Hohmann, E.L., Elde, R.P., Rysavy, J.A., Einzig, S., and Gebhard, R.L. (1986). Innervation of periosteum and bone by sympathetic vasoactive intestinal peptide-containing nerve fibers. *Science*, **232**, 868–71.

Honore, P., and Mantyh P.W. (2000). Bone cancer pain: from mechanism to model to therapy. *Pain Med.*, **1**, 303–9.

Honore, P., Luger, N.M., Sabino, M.A., *et al.* (2000a). Osteoprotegerin blocks bone cancer-induced skeletal destruction, skeletal pain and pain-related neurochemical reorganization of the spinal cord. *Nature Med.*, **6**, 521–8.

Honore, P., Menning, P.M., Rogers, S.D., Nichols, M.L., and Mantyh, P.W. (2000b). Neurochemical plasticity in persistent inflammatory pain. *Progr. Brain Res.*, **129**, 357–63.

Honore, P., Schwei, J., Rogers, S.D., *et al.* (2000c). Cellular and neurochemical remodeling of the spinal cord in bone cancer pain. *Progr. Brain Res.*, **129**, 389–97.

Hukkanen, M., Konttinen, Y.T., Rees, R.G., Gibson, S.J., Santavirta, S., and Polak, J.M. (1992). Innervation of bone from healthy and arthritic rats by substance P and calcitonin gene related peptide containing sensory fibers. *J. Rheumatol.*, **19**, 1252–9.

Lacey, D.L., Timms, E., Tan, H.L., *et al.* (1998). Osteoprotegerin ligand is a cytokine that regulates osteoclast differentiation and activation. *Cell*, **93**, 165–76.

Lassiter, L.K., and Carducci, M.A. (2003). Endothelin receptor antagonists in the treatment of prostate cancer. *Semin. Oncol.*, **30**, 678–88.

Ledeboer, A., Sloane, E.M., Milligan, E.D., *et al.* (2005). Minocycline attenuates mechanical allodynia and proinflammatory cytokine expression in rat models of pain facilitation. *Pain*, **115**, 71–83.

Luger, N.M., Honore, P., Sabino, M.A., *et al.* (2001). Osteoprotegerin diminishes advanced bone cancer pain. *Cancer Res.*, **61**, 4038–47.

Mach, D.B., Rogers, S.D., Sabino, M.C., *et al.* (2002). Origins of skeletal pain: sensory and sympathetic innervation of the mouse femur. *Neuroscience*, **113**, 155–66.

Mantyh, P.W. (2002). A mechanism based understanding of cancer pain. *Pain*, **96**, 1–2.

Mantyh, P.W., Clohisy, D.R., Koltzenburg, M., and Hunt, S.P. (2002). Molecular mechanisms of cancer pain. *Nature Rev. Cancer*, **2**, 201–9.

Medhurst, S.J., Walker, K., Bowes, M., *et al.* (2002). A rat model of bone cancer pain. *Pain*, **96**, 129–40.

13

Mocellin, S., Rossi, CR., Pilati, P., Nitti, D. (2005). Tumor necrosis factor, cancer and anticancer therapy. *Cytokine Growth Factor Rev.*, **16**, 35–53.

Murata, T., Ushikubi, F., Matsuoka, T., et al. (1997). Altered pain perception and inflammatory response in mice lacking prostacyclin receptor. *Nature*, **388**, 678–82.

Nelson, J.B., Hedican, S.P., George, D.J., et al. (1995). Identification of endothelin-1 in the pathophysiology of metastatic adenocarcinoma of the prostate. *Nature Med.*, **1**, 944–9.

North, R.A. (2002). Molecular physiology of P2X receptors. *Physiol, Rev.*, **82**, 1013–67.

Ogmundsdottir, H.M. (2001). Immune reaction to breast cancer: for better or for worse? *Archi. Immunol. Ther. Exp.*, **49** (Suppl. 2), S75–81.

Olson, T.H., Riedl, M.S., Vulchanova, L., Ortiz-Gonzalez, X.R. and Elde, R. (1998). An acid sensing ion channel (ASIC) localizes to small primary afferent neurons in rats. *Neuroreport*, **9**, 1109–13.

Portenoy, R.K., and Hagen, N.A. (1990). Breakthrough pain: definition, prevalence and characteristics. *Pain*, **41**, 273–81.

Reeh, P.W., and Steen, K.H. (1996). Tissue acidosis in nociception and pain. *Prog. Brain Res.*, **113**, 143–51.

Sabino, M.A., Luger, N.M., Mach, D.B., Rogers, S.D., Schwei, M.J. and Mantyh, P.W. (2003). Different tumors in bone each give rise to a distinct pattern of skeletal destruction, bone cancer-related pain behaviors and neurochemical changes in the central nervous system. *Int. J. Cancer*, **104**, 550–8.

Schmidt, R., Schmelz, M., Torebjork, H.E., and Handwerker, H.O. (2000). Mechano-insensitive nociceptors encode pain evoked by tonic pressure to human skin. *Neuroscience*, **98**, 793–800.

Schwei, M.J., Honore, P., Rogers, S.D., et al. (1999). Neurochemical and cellular reorganization of the spinal cord in a murine model of bone cancer pain. *J. Neuroscience*, **19**, 10886–97.

Serre, C.M., Farlay, D., Delmas, P.D., and Chenu, C. (1999). Evidence for a dense and intimate innervation of the bone tissue, including glutamate-containing fibers. *Bone*, **25**, 623–9.

Sevcik, M.A., Ghilardi, J.R., Peters, C.M., et al. (2005). Anti-NGF therapy profoundly reduces bone cancer pain and the accompanying increase in markers of peripheral and central sensitization. *Pain*, **115**, 128–41.

Sezer, O., Heider, U., Zavrski, I., Kuhne, C.A. and Hofbauer, L.C. (2003). RANK ligand and osteoprotegerin in myeloma bone disease. *Blood*, **101**, 2094–8.

Standal, T., Seidel, C., Hjertner, O., et al. (2002). Osteoprotegerin is bound, internalized, and degraded by multiple myeloma cells. *Blood*, **100**, 3002–7.

Suzuki, K. and Yamada, S. (1994). Ascites sarcoma 180, a tumor associated with hypercalcemia, secretes potent bone-resorbing factors including transforming growth factor alpha, interleukin-1 alpha and interleukin-6. *Bone Mineral*, **27**, 219–33.

Sweitzer, S.M., Schubert, P., and DeLeo, J.A. (2001). Propentofylline, a glial modulating agent, exhibits antiallodynic properties in a rat model of neuropathic pain. *J. Pharmacol. Exp. Therapeut.*, **297**, 1210–7.

Szczesny, G. (2002). Molecular aspects of bone healing and remodeling. *Polish J. Pathol.*, **53**, 145–53.

Takayanagi, H. (2005). Mechanistic insight into osteoclast differentiation in osteoimmunology. *J. Mol. Med.*, **83**, 170–9.

Thompson, S.W. and Tonge, D. (2000). Bone cancer gain without the pain. *Nature Med.*, **6**, 504–5.

Troen, B.R. (2003). Molecular mechanisms underlying osteoclast formation and activation. *Exp. Gerontol.*, **38**, 605–14.

Urch, C.E., Donovan-Rodriguez, T. and Dickenson, A.H. (2003). Alterations in dorsal horn neurones in a rat model of cancer-induced bone pain. *Pain*, **106**, 347–56.

Watkins, L.R., Milligan, E.D. and Maier, S.F. (2001). Glial activation: a driving force for pathological pain. *Trends Neurosci.*, **24**, 450–5.

Yasuda, H., Shima, N., Nakagawa, N., et al. (1998). Identity of osteoclastogenesis inhibitory factor (OCIF) and osteoprotegerin (OPG): a mechanism by which OPG/OCIF inhibits osteoclastogenesis *in vitro*. *Endocrinology*, **139**, 1329–37.

Zhang, R.X., Liu, B., Wang, L., et al. (2005). Spinal glial activation in a new rat model of bone cancer pain produced by prostate cancer cell inoculation of the tibia. *Pain*, **118**, 125–36.

16

Chapter 3

Clinical features

Marie T. Fallon and Sandra McConnell

3.1 Introduction

Bone pain is a significant clinical problem for patients, their carers and health care professionals. Thus, bone pain can have a significant impact on physical, psychological and social functioning (and so overall quality of life) (Rustoen et al., 2005). Furthermore, bone pain can be difficult to manage, and treatment may require the use of multiple types of intervention (Clare et al., 2005). This chapter will discuss the epidemiology, clinical features and relevance of bone pain in patients with cancer.

3.2 Epidemiology

Bone is the most common source of pain in patients with malignant disease (Twycross and Fairfield, 1982; Portenoy et al., 1999), with studies suggesting that ~28% of hospice inpatients (Loeser, 2000), 34% of patients in a cancer pain clinic (Banning et al., 1991), and 45% of advanced cancer patients followed up at home (Loeser, 2000) are affected by pain from bone metastases. Furthermore, studies suggest that lesions in bone account for 30–35% of all cancer pains in patients with advanced disease (Twycross and Fairfield, 1982; Grond et al., 1996).

Not everyone will have pain as a result of bone metastases. For example, one-third of patients with metastatic breast disease affecting the skeleton do not complain of pain (Front et al., 1979). However, other patients experience multiple pains. For example, in a study of cancer patients in Oxford, 31 patients complained of a total of 58 pains attributable to bone metastases (Twycross and Fairfield, 1982).

The presence of bone pain is independent of tumour type, location, number and size of metastases, gender and age of the patient (Oster et al., 1978).

3.3 **Clinical features**

Descriptors of cancer-related bone pain are varied, but it is generally accepted that there is a triad of background pain, spontaneous pain (a subtype of breakthrough pain) and incident pain (another subtype of breakthrough pain) (Mercadante and Arcuri, 1998; Urch, 2004).

Breakthrough pain refers to 'a transitory exacerbation of pain experienced by the patient who has relatively stable and adequately controlled baseline pain' (Portenoy et al., 2004). Spontaneous pain (also known as 'idiopathic pain') refers to episodes of breakthrough pain that occur unexpectedly. In contrast, incident pain (also known as 'precipitated pain' or, when appropriate, 'movement-related pain') refers to episodes of breakthrough pain that are related to specific events (Davies, 2006).

3.3.1 **Background pain**

Temporal pattern of pain

Background pain can be intermittent initially, but rapidly progresses to become constant in nature.

Site of pain

In a study where 41% of participants had pain due to neoplastic damage to bones and joints (Caraceni and Portenoy, 1999), 13% had vertebral (including sacral) pain, 7.1% had pelvic pain, 6.8% had pain in the chest wall from rib lesion(s), 3.9% had pain in the long bones and 10.2% had generalized bone pain from multiple bone metastases. The skeleton was affected in slightly different patterns depending on the primary site of the tumour (Table 3.1).

Radiation of pain

Usually the pain is localized to a specific area (and frequently there is point tenderness over the affected area of bone). In other cases, pain may be referred (Mercadante, 1997): for example, a metastatic deposit in the hip may result in pain in the knee area; a lesion in the T12/L1 site may cause pain felt in the iliac crest or sacro-iliac joint (either unilaterally or bilaterally); a cervical spine metastasis may have pain referred to the occipital region or the skull vertex (Loeser, 2000).

Another feature which is recognized in cancer-related bone pain is the phenomenon of a 'migratory pattern of pain', where pain might appear in one area of the body at a given time then move to a completely different part of the body with total resolution of the pain at the original site (Pollen and Schmidt, 1979).

Table 3.1 Prevalence of different pain syndromes in patients with different tumours (Caraceni and Portenoy, 1999)

Cancer diagnosis	Pain syndrome (%)					
	Skull	Vertebral	Pelvis and long bones	Generalised bone pain	Chest wall	Pathological fracture
All tumours	5.2	13.0	10.5	11.4	6.8	5.0
Breast	2.1	20.9	12.5	25.3	9.7	8.3
Lower GI tract	1.9	10.6	17.4	0	0.9	1.9
Upper GI tract	1.9	4.8	0.9	0.9	0	0
Head & neck	21.6	4.5	6.3	5.4	0.9	0.9
Leukaemia/lymphoma	0	4.7	11.9	14.2	0	0
Lung	4.6	18.0	8.8	10.4	20.7	7.7
Prostate	1.5	21.5	25.1	40.0	4.6	3.0
Uterus	0	4.2	4.2	0	2.8	0

Quality (character) of pain

Background pain is often described as a dull ache (Colleau, 2002). However, the descriptions of the pain were variable in a study of patients with bone pain from metastatic prostate cancer (Pollen and Schmidt, 1979).

Intensity (severity) of pain

The intensity of bone pain is independent of tumour type, location, number and size of metastases, gender and age of the patient (Oster et al., 1978).

In a study of patients with bone pain from metastatic prostate cancer, 60% had 'severe' pain, 30% had 'moderate' pain, and the rest described their pain as being 'mild' (Pollen and Schmidt, 1979). Bone pain usually increases in intensity over time (Mercadante, 1997).

Interestingly, a study of hospitalized patients with advanced cancer demonstrated that, while 49% of patients with bone metastases reported severe pain, only 31% of patients without bone involvement reported a similar level of pain (Brescia et al., 1990).

Exacerbating factors of pain

As discussed above, exacerbations of pain may be related to specific events ('incident pain'). Incident pain can be further divided into: (a) volitional pain—precipitated by a voluntary act, e.g. walking; (b) non-volitional—precipitated by an involuntary act, e.g. coughing (Davies, 2006).

Relieving factors of pain

A variety of different non-pharmacological, pharmacological, oncological and other types of interventions have been used to treat bone pain. These interventions are discussed in detail in the subsequent chapters.

Other features of pain

As bone pain due to cancer becomes more established, mechanical allodynia can develop, resulting in pain from a stimulus or activity which is normally not painful e.g. coughing, moving in bed (Clohisy and Mantyh, 2003).

Recent studies also suggest that cancer-related bone pain can result in paraesthesia (altered sensation), dynamic allodynia (perception of pain in response to light brushing of the skin), static allodynia (perception of pain in response to pressure), or thermal hyperalgesia (pain at normal, low and high temperature thresholds)[AD1] (Medhurst et al., 2002: Menendez et al., 2003).

3.3.2 **Breakthrough pain**

An International Association for the Study of Pain (IASP) survey found that breakthrough pain was present according to clinicians in 65% of patients with cancer-related pain (Caraceni and Portenoy,

1999; Caraceni et al., 2004). However, breakthrough pain was more likely to be reported in English-speaking countries, which may reflect factors to do with the definition, or the recognition, of the phenomenon.

Bone pain is a major source of breakthrough pain, and is the predominant source of incident pain (Caraceni et al., 2004). In the aforementioned survey, breakthrough pain was significantly associated with certain pain syndromes, including those due to vertebral lesions, and lesions in the pelvis, long bones or joints. Thus, of the patients with vertebral pain syndrome, 85% had breakthrough pain. Similarly, of the patients with pelvis and long bone lesions, 78% had breakthrough pain.

The clinical features of breakthrough pain vary from individual to individual (Portenoy et al., 2004). Nevertheless, breakthrough pain is often reported to be frequent in occurrence, acute in onset, short in duration, and moderate-to-severe in intensity (Portenoy and Hagen, 1990; Portenoy et al., 1999; Zeppetella et al., 2000). For example, Zeppetella et al., (2000) reported a mean number of four episodes per day (range 0–14 episodes per day) among hospice inpatients with pain. Similarly, Portenoy et al., (1999) found the median interval between onset and peak of pain to be 3 min, with a range of 1 sec–30 min. In addition, Portenoy and Hagen (1990) reported a median duration of 30 min (range 1–240 min) amongst hospital inpatients with pain. The clinical features of breakthrough pain often mirror the clinical features of the background pain.

The clinical features of breakthrough pain may also vary within an individual. For example, patients may experience both spontaneous pain and incident pain. In the study by Portenoy et al., (1999), almost two-thirds of patients could identify a precipitant for their pain, such as weight-bearing and/or movement. However, nearly half of patients also stated that their pain could be unpredictable at times.

Patients with breakthrough pain have more intense background pain than those without breakthrough pain (Portenoy et al., 1999; Caraceni et al., 2004). Moreover, the study by Portenoy et al., (1999) confirms that patients with breakthrough pain have greater functional impairment (as measured on the interference scale of the Brief Pain Inventory) when compared to patients without such pain. In addition, patients with breakthrough pain have significantly increased levels of depression and anxiety (as measured by the Beck Depression Inventory and the Beck Anxiety Inventory) when compared with patients without such pain.

It should be noted that the aforementioned data are derived from studies involving patients with all types of cancer pain, and that to date there are no published studies involving patients with solely bone pain.

3.3.3 **Complications of bone pain**

Cancer-related bone pain is associated with physical morbidity, psychological morbidity (anxiety, depression), reduced performance status, and impaired quality of life (Portenoy et al., 1999). Furthermore, cancer-related bone pain is associated with a variety of social problems: patients with bone pain often find that their work and leisure activities are adversely affected by their pain (Coward and Wilkie, 2000).

In addition, family relationships are sometimes strained when the pain reduces the patients' tolerance of others. Indeed, some patients cope with their pain by isolating themselves, which can lead to further difficulties (Coward and Wilkie, 2000). Similarly, some patients prefer not to tell anyone about their pain (Coward and Wilkie, 2000).

In a small descriptive study of patients with metastatic bone disease, pain was regarded by the patients as a metaphor for cancer and its recurrence (Coward and Wilkie, 2000). Thus, patients were frightened that pain meant that previous cancer treatments had been ineffective, and, as a result, they were uncertain about whether the cancer could be controlled. However, pain was also perceived as protective, by encouraging patients to seek more cancer treatment, and by encouraging the prevention of 'doing too much' and so causing further harm.

3.3.4 **Other complications of bone disease**

In addition to pain, bone metastases can result in several other serious problems including pathological fracture, neurological complications (such as nerve or spinal cord compression), bone marrow suppression, hypercalcaemia, deep vein thrombosis, and pulmonary embolism. Each of these problems has a detrimental effect on patients' quality of life.

Pathological fracture

Pathological fracture, secondary to increased bone fragility, occurs in 8–30% of patients with bone metastases (Mercadante, 1997). The likelihood of pathological fracture increases with the duration of metastatic involvement. Thus, it is higher in patients in whom metastases are confined to the skeleton, and in those patients who have an otherwise relatively good prognosis.

Fracture is common in osteolytic bone lesions and is, therefore, more likely in patients with breast carcinoma and myeloma. In one study it was reported that the median time for women with stage IV breast cancer who were receiving chemotherapy, and had at least one lytic bone metastasis, to have a major skeletal event (i.e. pathological fracture, or need for radiotherapy/orthopaedic surgery, or spinal cord compression, or hypercalcaemia) was 7 months (Hortobagyi et al., 1996).

Long bones are frequently involved, but vertebral collapse is even more common (Paterson et al., 1991).

The risk of pathological fracture through a bone metastasis can be assessed using Mirels' scale, which is a scoring system combining radiographic and clinical features (see Table 10.1) (Mirels, 1989). Site (upper limb, lower limb, or peritrochanteric), pain intensity (mild, moderate, or functional), type of lesion (blastic, lytic, or mixed) and size of metastasis on radiograph are noted to give a total score, and indicate the risk of fracture/need for surgical fixation. Pain aggravated by function, and lesions measuring more than two thirds of the diameter of the bone, are major predictors of impending fractures (Mirels, 1989).

Neurological complications

Nerve compression can occur where nerves lie adjacent to affected bone. This can cause neuropathic pain and/or other neurological problems. The most serious complication is one of spinal cord compression.

Spinal cord compression is usually the result of the growth of metastatic deposits in the vertebral bodies: if the lesion grows posteriorly, and extends into the epidural space, pressure is exerted on the spinal cord causing mechanical injury. In addition, compression of its vascular supply may result in ischaemia, venous stasis and infarction. As a consequence of these changes, progressive neurological deficits develop distal to the site of the compression, e.g. compressive lesions in the cervical vertebrae cause tetraplegia, those in the thoracic vertebrae cause paraplegia, and those in the lumbar region precipitate the cauda equina syndrome.

The onset of neurological symptoms is often insidious, although once neurological symptoms have become established they tend to develop rapidly. Typically, there is radicular pain (unilateral in cervical and lumbosacral involvement, and bilateral in thoracic involvement). Neck flexion, straight leg raising, recumbency, coughing and local pressure frequently exacerbate the pain, whereas sitting up or lying very still may bring relief from pain. Muscle weakness, sphincter impairment and sensory loss are unusual in the early stages, but develop as the compression progresses.

Early detection and treatment significantly improve the functional outcome in spinal cord compression (Ingham et al., 1993).

Bone marrow suppression

As bone metastases generally affect the areas of the skeleton where red marrow is located, widespread disease can cause bone marrow suppression (and therefore symptoms/signs of anaemia, infection and bleeding).

23

Hypercalcaemia

It is estimated that 5–10% of all cancer patients are affected by hypercalcaemia during their illness (Coleman, 1997). Hypercalcaemia is particularly common in breast cancer, multiple myeloma, squamous carcinoma of the lung and other sites (Coleman, 1997), affecting up to one-third of those patients with advanced disease (Lamy and Burckhardt, 2002). However, hypercalcaemia does not correlate with the extent of metastatic bone disease, and can occur in the absence of bone metastases (Lamy et al., 2001).

Deep vein thrombosis/pulmonary embolism

Many patients with bone disease find movement so unpleasant that they become progressively more immobile, which increases their risk of deep vein thrombosis and pulmonary embolism. It should be noted that these complications are already common as a result of the prothrombotic state associated with malignancy.

Other complications

Other complications are rare, and include those due to cancer treatment such as osteonecrosis either as a result of radiotherapy or corticosteroid use (Portenoy and Lesage, 1999).

3.3.5 **Natural history**

Bone metastases invariably signify advanced/incurable disease. Once bone metastases have been identified, the average life expectancy for patients with breast carcinoma is 34 months (range 1–90 months) (Koenders et al., 1992), for patients with prostate carcinoma (who are under 65 years of age) is 24 months (Lote et al., 1986), and for patients with lung cancer is <12 months (Nielsen et al., 1991). However, the median survivals are much less: for example, breast cancer patients have a median survival of 33 months (48 months for those in whom the disease is confined to the skeleton, and 9 months for those with additional visceral metastases) (Sherry et al., 1986).

References

Banning, A., Sjogren, P. and Henriksen, H. (1991). Pain causes in 200 patients referred to a multidisciplinary cancer pain clinic. Pain, **45**, 45–8.

Brescia, F.J., Adler, D., Gray, G., Ryan, M.A., Cimino, J., and Mamtani, R. (1990). Hospitalized advanced cancer patients: a profile. J. Pain Sympt. Management, **5**, 221–7.

Caraceni, A., and Portenoy, R.K. (1999). An international survey of cancer pain characteristics and syndromes. Pain, **82**, 263–74.

Caraceni, A., Martini, C., Zecca, E., et al. (2004). Breakthrough pain characteristics and syndromes in patients with cancer pain. An international survey. Palliat. Med., **18**, 177–83.

Clare, C., Royle, D., Saharia, K., Pearse, H., Oxberry, S., Oakley, K. et al. (2005). Painful bone metastases: a prospective observational cohort study. Palliat. Med., 19, 521–5.

Clohisy, D.R., and Mantyh, P.W. (2003). Bone cancer pain. Clin. Orthop. Related Res., (415 Suppl), S279–88.

Coleman, R.E. (1997). Skeletal complications of malignancy. Cancer, 80, 1588–94.

Colleau, S.M. (2002). Palliation of bone pain in cancer: facts and controversies. Cancer Pain Release, 15, 1.

Coward, D.D., and Wilkie, D.J. (2000). Metastatic bone pain: meanings associated with self-report and self-management decision making. Cancer Nursing, 23, 101–8.

Davies, A.N. (2006). Introduction. In Davies, A.N. (ed.) Cancer-related breakthrough pain, pp. 1–11. Oxford University Press, Oxford.

Front, D., Schneck, S.O., Frankel, A., and Robinson, E. (1979). Bone metastases and bone pain in breast cancer. JAMA, 242, 1747–8.

Grond, S., Zech, D., Diefenbach, C., Radbruch, L., and Lehmann, K.A. (1996). Assessment of cancer pain: a prospective evaluation in 2266 cancer patients referred to a pain service. Pain, 64, 107–14.

Hortobagyi, G.N., Theriault, R.L., Porter, L., Blayney, D., Lipton, A., Sinoff, C. et al. (1996). Efficacy of pamidronate in reducing skeletal complications in patients with breast cancer and lytic bone metastases. Protocol 19 Aredia Breast Study Group. New Engl. J. Med., 335, 1785–91.

Ingham, J., Beveridge, A., and Cooney, N.J. (1993). The management of spinal cord compression in patients with advanced malignancy. J. Pain Sympt. Management, 8, 1–6.

Koenders, P.G., Beex, L.V., Kloppenborg, P.W., Smals, A.G., and Benraad, T.J. (1992). Human breast cancer: survival from first metastasis. Breast Cancer Study Group. Breast Cancer Res. Treatment, 21, 173–80.

Lamy, O., and Burckhardt, P. (2002). Hypercalcaemia of malignancy: diagnosis and treatment options. Am. J. Cancer, 1, 277–92.

Lamy, O., Jenzer-Closuit, A., and Burckhardt, P. (2001). Hypercalcaemia of malignancy: an undiagnosed and undertreated disease. J. Intern. Med., 250, 73–9.

Loeser, J.D. (2000). Cancer pain: assessment and diagnosis. In Bonica, J.J., and Loeser, J.D., (ed). Bonica's management of pain, pp. 634–41. Lippincott/Williams K Wilkins, Philadelphia.[AD2]

Lote, K., Walloe, A., and Bjersand, A., (1986). Bone metastasis, Prognosis, diagnosis and treatment Acta Radiol. Oncol. 25, 227–32.

Medhurst, S.J., Walker, K., Bowes, M. et al. (2002). A rat model of bone cancer pain. Pain 96, 129–40.

Menendez, L., Lastra, A., Fresno, M.F. et al. (2003). Initial thermal heat hypoalgesia and delayed hyperalgesia in a murine model of bone cancer pain. Brain Res. 969, 102–9.

Mercadante, S. (1997). Malignant bone pain: pathophysiology and treatment. Pain, 69, 1–18.

Mercadante, S., and Arcuri, E. (1998). Breakthrough pain in cancer patients: pathophysiology and treatment. *Cancer Treatment Rev.*, **24**, 425–32.

Mirels, H. (1989). Metastatic disease in long bones. A proposed scoring system for diagnosing impending pathological fractures. *Clin. Orthop. Related Res.*, **249**, 256–64.

Nielsen, O.S., Munro, A.J., and Tannock, I.F. (1991). Bone metastases: pathophysiology and management policy. *J. Clin. Oncol.*, **9**, 509–24.

Oster, M.W., Vizel, M., and Turgeon, L.R. (1978). Pain of terminal cancer patients. *Arch Intern. Med.*, **138**, 1801–2.

Paterson, A.H., Ernst, D.S., Powles, T.J., Ashley, S., McCloskey, E.V., and Kanis, J.A. (1991). Treatment of skeletal disease in breast cancer with clodronate. *Bone*, **12** (Suppl. 1), S25–30.

Pollen, J.J., and Schmidt, J.D. (1979). Bone pain in metastatic cancer of prostate. *Urology*, **13**, 129–34.

Portenoy, R.K., Forbes, K., Lussier, D., and Hanks, G. (2004). Difficult pain problems: an integrated approach. In Doyle D, Hanks G, Cherny N, and Calman K, (ed.) *Oxford textbook of palliative medicine* (3rd edn), pp. 438–58. Oxford University Press, Oxford.

Portenoy, R.K., and Hagen, N.A. (1990). Breakthrough pain: definition, prevalence and characteristics. *Pain*, **41**, 273–81.

Portenoy, R.K., and Lesage, P. (1999). Management of cancer pain. *Lancet*, **353**, 1695–700.

Portenoy, R.K., Payne, D., and Jacobsen, P. (1999). Breakthrough pain: characteristics and impact in patients with cancer pain. *Pain*, **81**, 129–34.

Rustoen, T., Moum, T., Padilla, G., Paul, S., and Miaskowski, C. (2005). Predictors of quality of life in oncology outpatients with pain from bone metastasis. *J. Pain Sympt. Management*, **30**, 234–42.

Sherry, M.M., Greco, F.A., Johnson, D.H., and Hainsworth, J.D. (1986). Metastatic breast cancer confined to the skeletal system. An indolent disease. *Am. J. Med.*, **81**, 381–6.

Twycross, R.G., and Fairfield, S. (1982). Pain in far-advanced cancer. *Pain*, **14**, 303–10.

Urch, C. (2004). The pathophysiology of cancer-induced bone pain: current understanding. *Palliat. Med.*, **18**, 267–74.

Zeppetella, G., O'Doherty, C.A., and Collins, S. (2000). Prevalence and characteristics of breakthrough pain in cancer patients admitted to a hospice. *J. Pain Sympt. Management*, **20**, 87–92.

Chapter 4

General principles of management

Andrew Davies

4.1 Introduction

The successful management of bone pain depends on adequate assessment, appropriate treatment, and adequate reassessment (i.e. assessment of the treatment) (Davies, 2002). Inadequate assessment may lead to ineffective treatment, or even inappropriate treatment. Similarly, inadequate reassessment may lead to continuance of ineffective/inappropriate treatment (and continuance of pain).

This chapter will discuss the assessment of bone pain, and the general principles of management of bone pain. Subsequent chapters will discuss the radiological investigation (Chapter 5), oncological management (Chapter 8), pharmacological management (Chapters 6 and 7), interventional pain management (Chapter 9), and orthopaedic surgical management (Chapter 10), of bone pain in more detail.

4.2 Assessment

The assessment of bone pain primarily depends on basic clinical skills, i.e. taking a history and performing an examination (Davies, 2002). It is important to take a general history, as well as a pain history. In particular, patients should be screened for psychological, spiritual, and social factors that may be contributing to their experience of pain (the concept of 'total pain') (Twycross, 1994). Similarly, it is important to perform a general examination, as well as an examination of the painful area. Radiological investigations can be extremely useful in the assessment of bone pain (see Chapter 5). Nevertheless, radiological investigations should only be viewed as a part of the assessment process, rather than the main focus of the assessment process. Thus, investigations may produce both false negative results, and false positive results.

Many patients with bone pain experience a combination of background pain [a 'constant or continuous pain of long duration' (Ferrell et al., 1999)], and of breakthrough pain ['a transitory exacerbation of pain experienced by the patient who has relatively stable and adequately controlled baseline pain' (Portenoy et al., 2004)]. Although there is often a close relationship between these different types of pain (Portenoy et al., 1999), it is important that they are individually assessed, and, where necessary, individually managed (Davies, 2006).

4.2.1 **History**

All patients require a detailed pain history to be taken. The features of the pain that need to be determined include (Foley, 2004):

- onset
- temporal pattern
- site
- radiation
- quality (i.e. character)
- intensity (i.e. severity)—it is important to determine the baseline pain intensity, as this will serve as a marker of the response to treatment
- exacerbating factors
- relieving factors
- response to analgesics
- response to other interventions (e.g. anticancer treatment, non-pharmacological interventions)
- associated physical symptoms
- associated psychological symptoms
- interference with activities of daily living—it is important to determine the baseline impact of pain, as this can also serve a marker of the response to treatment.

4.2.2 **Examination**

All patients require a thorough examination to be performed. It can be useful to reproduce the patient's pain by using so-called 'provocative manoeuvres' (e.g. palpation, passive movement) (Hagen, 1999). However, it is important that the benefits of such manoeuvres (i.e. improved understanding of the pain) outweigh the costs of these manoeuvres (i.e. causation of the pain). The examination should include a neurological examination, since the presence of neurological signs may suggest an associated neurological complication (e.g. nerve root compression, spinal cord compression.

4.3 **Treatment**

The management of bone pain is highly individualized, and may involve one or more of the following strategies:

- treatment of the underlying cancer
- treatment of the underlying pathology (e.g. resorption of bone, fracture of bone)
- symptomatic treatment of the background pain
- symptomatic treatment of any breakthrough pain
- treatment of the complications (e.g. nerve root compression, spinal cord compression).

A number of factors will influence the management strategy, including disease-related factors (e.g. tumour stage), patient-related factors (e.g. performance status), and the availability of relevant resources.

4.3.1 **Treatment of underlying cancer**

The optimal treatment for the cancer is somewhat dependent on the type of cancer. Nevertheless, radiotherapy can be effective in treating bone metastases from a variety of different types of cancer (Hoskin, 2004). Furthermore, radiotherapy provides significant pain relief within a relatively short period of time (in contrast to other treatment modalities that may not provide significant pain relief for several months). The role of radiotherapy in the management of bone pain is discussed in more detail in Chapter 8.

4.3.2 **Treatment of underlying pathology**

Bisphosphonates are an established treatment of cancer-related bone disease (Krempien et al., 2005): they are used to treat established disease, as well as to prevent the development of new disease. Analgesic effects may be seen soon after the initiation of the treatment, although major analgesic effects are only seen after several months of the treatment (i.e. after 'healing' of the bone). Bisphosphonates are discussed in more detail in Chapter 7.

In some cases of fracture/impending fracture, it may be appropriate to perform surgical stabilization of the relevant bone(s) (see Chapter 10). Alternatively, in other cases, it may be possible to use an orthotic device to stabilize the relevant bone(s) (Figure 4.1) (Mercadante and Arcuri, 1998). Moreover, many patients will benefit from strategies to minimize the amount of movement required, such as provision of simple adaptations to their surroundings, and provision of additional practical support with the activities of daily living (Mercadante and Arcuri, 1998).

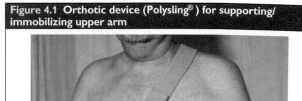

Figure 4.1 Orthotic device (Polysling®) for supporting/immobilizing upper arm

4.3.3 Symptomatic treatment of background pain

The symptomatic treatment of bone pain is based on guidelines produced by the World Health Organization (1996). The guidelines cover all aspects of the management of pain, although they focus on the pharmacological management of pain; the guidelines promote five main principles with regard to the pharmacological management of pain:

1. 'By mouth'—drugs should be given orally (if possible).
2. 'By the clock'—drugs should be given regularly.
3. 'By the ladder'—drugs are given in a stepwise manner (Figure 4.2).
4. 'For the individual'—opioid drugs should be individually titrated.
5. 'Attention to detail'.

The role of non-opioids, opioids for mild to moderate pain, and opioids for moderate to severe pain is discussed in detail in Chapter 6. Bisphosphonates are considered to be adjuvant analgesics for bone pain (see above), and there is some animal data to suggest that certain drugs for neuropathic pain may also be useful adjuvant analgesics for bone pain (e.g. gabapentin) (Donovan-Rodriguez et al., 2005). Corticosteroids may also have a role to play in this type of pain (Hanks, 1988).

A variety of non-pharmacological techniques has been used to treat bone pain, including rubbing/massage, application of heat, application of cold, transcutaneous nerve stimulation (TENS), acupuncture, distraction techniques, and relaxation techniques. However, the evidence base for these techniques in the management of bone pain is somewhat limited. Similarly, a variety of interventional techniques has been used to treat refractory bone pain (see Chapter 9).

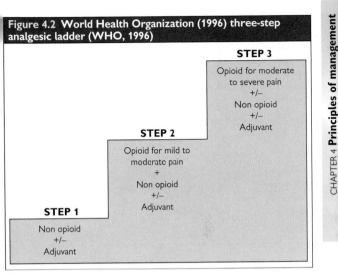

Figure 4.2 World Health Organization (1996) three-step analgesic ladder (WHO, 1996)

STEP 3
Opioid for moderate
to severe pain
+/–
Non opioid
+/–
Adjuvant

STEP 2
Opioid for mild to
moderate pain
+
Non opioid
+/–
Adjuvant

STEP 1
Non opioid
+/–
Adjuvant

4.3.4 **Symptomatic treatment of breakthrough pain**

Breakthrough pain is not a single entity, but a spectrum of very different entities. For example, patients with bone pain may experience spontaneous pain (breakthrough pain that occurs unexpectedly), incident pain (breakthrough pain that is related to specific events), or a combination of the two types of pain. The management of breakthrough pain is often different from that of background pain, and the management of spontaneous pain is often different from that of incident pain. Indeed, the management of breakthrough pain is highly individualized (Patt and Ellison, 1998).

The symptomatic treatment of breakthrough pain includes (Davies, 2006):

- Pharmacological treatment of pain:
  1. Modification of the background analgesic regimen
     (a) increase dose of analgesic drugs;
     (b) addition of analgesic drugs;
     (c) addition of co-analgesic drugs.
  2. Use of breakthrough ('rescue') analgesics
     (a) non-opioid analgesics;
     (b) opioid analgesics;
     (c) other agents, e.g. nitrous oxide, midazolam.
- Non-pharmacological treatment of pain (see above).

The management of breakthrough pain is discussed in more detail in Chapter 6.

4.4 **Reassessment procedure**

The primary objective of reassessment is to determine the efficacy and tolerability of any therapeutic intervention. A further objective of reassessment is the identification of significant changes in the pain. For example, increasing pain in a bone may represent impending fracture of that bone (which may necessitate a more intensive therapeutic intervention e.g. surgical stabilisation).

Various outcome measures have been used to assess the efficacy of therapeutic interventions, including (Davies, 2002):

- intensity of pain
- distress of pain
- pain relief
- satisfaction with treatment
- improvement in function
- improvement in quality of life.

The different outcome measures relate to different aspects of the pain. Consequently, there is often a poor correlation between the results obtained with different outcome measures. For example, in one study involving oncology patients, the percentage of subjects that were 'inadequately treated' varied from 16 to 91% depending on the specific outcome measure used (deWit et al., 1999).

All of the aforementioned outcome measures have limitations. For example, pain relief is related to the change in pain intensity over a period of time, i.e. it is dependent on the patient's recollection of the baseline pain intensity. There is little consensus on the specific outcome measure that should be used to assess treatment response (deWit et al., 1999). Nevertheless, it is important that a (suitable) outcome measure is used to assess treatment response in all patients (Davies, 2002).

Outcome measures are usually based on either a verbal rating scale, a numerical rating scale, or a visual analogue scale (Figure 4.3). Studies have shown a good correlation between the results obtained with these different scales (McQuay and Moore, 1998): the relationship between the results obtained with these different scales is shown in Table 4.1. However, patients with advanced cancer often have difficulty in completing such outcome measures. For example, in one study involving palliative care inpatients, 45% of the subjects were unable to complete any of the outcome measures (mainly because of cognitive impairment) (Shannon et al., 1995).

Figure 4.3 Examples of pain measurement scales

- Verbal rating scale, e.g. McGill Pain Questionnaire (Melzack, 1975).

  No pain; mild; discomforting; distressing; horrible; excruciating

- Numerical rating scale, e.g. Brief Pain Inventory (Daut et al., 1983).

  A. Pain intensity

  0   1   2   3   4   5   6   7   8   9   10

  No   Pain as bad
  pain   as you can
                                                 imagine

  B. Pain relief

  0% 10% 20% 30% 40% 50% 60% 70% 80% 90% 100%

  No   Complete
  relief   relief

- Visual anologue scale, e.g. Memorial Pain Assessment Card (Fishman et al., 1987).

  A. Pain intensity

  LEAST   **WORST**
  possible   ——————————————————————   possible
  pain   pain

  B. Pain relief

  NO   **COMPLETE**
  relief   ——————————————————————   relief
  of pain   of pain

Table 4.1 Correlation between results of different pain measurement scales

Verbal rating scale	Numerical rating scale (0–10)[*]	Visual analogue scale (100 mm)[+]
None	0	–
Mild	1–4	–
Moderate	5–6	>30 mm (mean 49)
Severe	7–10	>54 mm (mean 75)

[*] Serlin et al. (1995).

[+] Collins et al. (1997).

In addition to the aforementioned unidimensional pain assessment tools, there are a number of multidimensional pain assessment tools that have been validated in patients with cancer, e.g. Brief Pain Inventory (long and short form) (Daut et al., 1983), the McGill Pain Questionnaire (long and short form) (Melzack, 1975), and the Memorial Pain Assessment Card (Fishman et al., 1987). These tools are generally used in the research setting, rather than in the clinical setting.

Studies suggest that the formal measurement of pain leads to the improved management of pain. For example, in one study involving oncology outpatients, subjects whose outcome measures were reviewed were more likely to have had an improvement in their background pain intensity at follow-up than subjects whose outcome measures were unavailable for review (Trowbridge et al., 1997).

References

Collins, S.L., Moore, A., and McQuay, H.J. (1997). The visual analogue pain intensity scale: what is moderate pain in millimetres? *Pain*, **72**, 95–7.

Daut, R.L., Cleeland, C.S., and Flanery, R.C. (1983). Development of the Wisconsin Brief Pain Questionnaire to assess pain in cancer and other diseases. *Pain*, **17**, 197–210.

Davies, A. (2002). The assessment and measurement of physical pain. In: Hillier, R., Finlay, I., Miles, A. (ed.) *The effective management of cancer pain* (2nd edn), pp. 23–8. Aesculapius Medical Press, London.

Davies, A. (2006). General principles of management. In: Davies, A. (ed.) *Cancer-related breakthrough pain*. Oxford University Press, Oxford.

de Wit R, van Dam F, Abu-Saad HH et al. (1999). Empirical comparison of commonly used measures to evaluate pain treatment in cancer patients with chronic pain. *J. Clin. Oncol.*, **17**, 1280–7.

Donovan-Rodriguez, T., Dickenson, A.H., and Urch, C.E. (2005). Gabapentin normalizes spinal neuronal responses that correlate with behavior in a rat model of cancer-induced bone pain. *Anesthesiology*, **102**, 132–40.

Ferrell, B.R., Juarez, G., and Borneman, T. (1999). Use of routine and breakthrough analgesia in home care. *Oncol. Nursing Forum*, **26**, 1655–61.

Fishman, B., Pasternak, S., Wallenstein, S.L., Houde, R.W., Holland, J.C., and Foley K.M. (1987). The Memorial Pain Assessment Card: a valid instrument for the evaluation of cancer pain. *Cancer*, **60**, 1151–8.

Foley, K.M. (2004). Acute and chronic cancer pain syndromes. In: Doyle, D., Hanks, G., Cherny, N., and Calman, K. (ed.) *Oxford textbook of palliative medicine* (3rd edn), pp. 298–316. Oxford University Press, Oxford.

Hagen, N.A. (1999). Reproducing a cancer patient's pain on physical examination: bedside provocative maneuvers. *J. Pain Symptom Management*, **18**, 406–11.

Hanks, G.W. (1988). The pharmacological treatment of bone pain. *Cancer Surv.*, **7**, 87–101.

Hoskin, P.J. (2004). Radiotherapy in symptom management. In Doyle, D., Hanks, G., Cherny, N., Calman, K. (ed.) *Oxford textbook of palliative medicine* (3rd edn), pp. 239–55. Oxford University Press, Oxford.

Krempien, R., Niethammer, A., Harms, W., and Debus, J. (2005). Bisphosphonates and bone metastases: current status and future directions. Expert Rev. Anticancer Ther., **5**, 295–305.

McQuay, H.J., and Moore, R.A. (1998). *An evidence-based resource for pain relief.* Oxford University Press, Oxford.

Melzack, R. (1975). The McGill Pain Questionnaire: major properties and scoring methods. *Pain*, **1**, 277–99.

Mercadante, S., and Arcuri, E. (1998). Breakthrough pain in cancer patients: pathophysiology and treatment. *Cancer Treatment Rev.*, **24**, 425–32.

Patt, R.B., and Ellison, N.M. (1998). Breakthrough pain in cancer patients: characteristics, prevalence, and treatment. *Oncology (Huntington)*, **12**, 1035–52.

Portenoy, R.K., Forbes, K., Lussier, D., and Hanks, G. (2004). Difficult pain problems: an integrated approach. In: Doyle, D., Hanks, G., Cherny, N., Calman, K. (ed.) *Oxford textbook of palliative medicine* (3rd edn), pp. 438–58. Oxford University Press, Oxford.

Portenoy, R.K., Payne, D., and Jacobsen, P. (1999). Breakthrough pain: characteristics and impact in patients with cancer pain. *Pain*, **81**, 129–34.

Serlin, R.C., Mendoza, T.R., Nakamura, Y., Edwards, K.R., and Cleeland, C.S. (1995). When is cancer pain mild, moderate or severe? Grading pain severity by its interference with function. *Pain*, **61**, 277–84.

Shannon, M.M., Ryan, M.A., D'Agostino, N., and Brescia, F.J. (1995). Assessment of pain in advanced cancer patients. *J. Pain Symptom Management*, **10**, 274–8.

Trowbridge, R., Dugan, W., Jay, S.J. et al. (1997). Determining the effectiveness of a clinical-practice intervention in improving the control of pain in outpatients with cancer. *Acad. Med.*, **72**, 798–800.

Twycross, R. (1994). *Pain relief in advanced cancer.* Churchill Livingstone, Edinburgh.

World Health Organization (1996). *Cancer pain relief* (2nd edn). World Health Organization, Geneva.

Chapter 5

Radiology

David MacVicar and James Crawshaw

5.1 Introduction

The primary tumours that are notorious for metastasizing to bone are lung, breast, prostate, kidney and thyroid tumours, although any tumour can spread to bone apart from the primary brain (glial) tumours. Most bone metastases occur in the axial or proximal appendicular skeleton, but they may also occur in peripheral bones such as those of the hands and feet (e.g. lung tumours, melanoma). Bone metastases are typically multiple, although ~10% are solitary (e.g. lung tumours, kidney tumours).

Imaging plays the central role in the detection of bone metastases, and this chapter will discuss the strengths and weaknesses of the various imaging techniques used to identify such metastases. Imaging also plays a role in the management of bone metastases, particularly in terms of facilitating interventional techniques, such as percutaneous vertebral cementoplasty, percutaneous balloon kyphoplasty, and direct bone tumour ablation (e.g. radiofrequency ablation, cryoablation). These interventional techniques are discussed in detail in Chapter 9.

5.2 Plain film radiography

The principle of image production relies on the differential absorption of X-radiation by various tissues in the body. The atomic number and the electron density of elements are the key physical properties that allow discrimination of one tissue from another. Bone contains a significant amount of calcium, which has a high atomic number and a high electron density, and so absorbs much of the radiation that passes through it (as opposed to the surrounding soft tissues).

Plain film radiography remains an extremely valuable method of assessing bone pain. If a patient with cancer develops pain, then it is an entirely reasonable strategy to commence investigation with a radiograph of the part that is painful. However, it should be remembered that pain may be referred (e.g. a lesion at the ankle may cause pain towards the knee).

The typical features of a malignant lesion include abnormality of the trabecular pattern of the bone, and abnormal density of the bone (either reduced for a lytic deposit, or increased for a sclerotic deposit) (Figures 5.1 and 5.2). There is usually a wide zone of transition between a malignant lesion and the surrounding normal bone (cf. a narrow zone of transition between a benign lesion and the surrounding normal bone) (Figure 5.3), and there may be a periosteal reaction and/or an associated soft tissue mass.

The strengths of plain film radiography lie in it being readily available, speedy to perform, and that the features of malignant bony lesions are well described and widely recognized. The disadvantage of plain film radiography is its insensitivity (compared to other imaging techniques). Thus, at least 50% of cortical bone must be destroyed before a lesion becomes apparent on plain film radiography (Edelstyn et al., 1967).

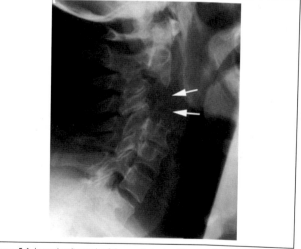

Figure 5.1 Lateral radiograph of the cervical spine. The vertebral bodies of C3 and C4 have been replaced by lytic metastatic disease from a renal cell carcinoma (arrows).

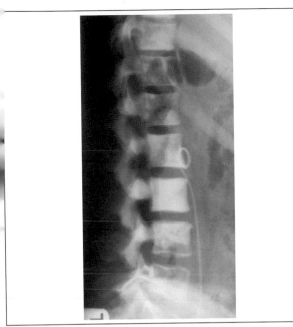

Figure 5.2 Lateral radiograph of the lumbar spine in a patient with metastatic carcinoma of the prostate. Some of the bones are extremely dense (e.g. L3). Elsewhere there is variable density of bone, indicating co-existing lytic and sclerotic metastatic disease.

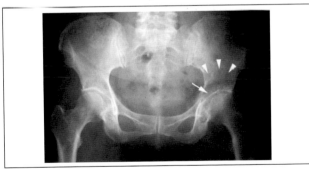

Figure 5.3 Plain radiograph of the pelvis performed for left hip pain in a patient with carcinoma of the breast. There is a diffuse lytic deposit in the left iliac bone extending to the acetabular roof. Note the destruction of normal bony trabeculae in the left acetabulum (white arrow). Normal bony trabeculae can be identified superior to the right acetabulum. There is a wide and indistinct zone of transition between the metastasis and the surrounding normal bone (arrowheads).

5.3 **Computed tomography (CT)**

A component of modern CT practice is the 'bony window review'. Moreover, the modern multi-slice CT scanners with spiral technique are capable of producing coronal, sagittal and three-dimensional re-formats to facilitate the imaging of specific regions.

CT is more sensitive than plain film radiography in detecting tumour within bone. It is also useful for assessing fractures in greater detail, and for detecting soft tissue masses associated with bone disease (Figure 5.5).

However, CT suffers from a relative lack of sensitivity in that fairly extensive marrow disease may be present but not detectable (Figure 5.6). Isotope studies and magnetic resonance imaging have a greater sensitivity for detection of bone metastases (see below).

5.4 **Bone scintigraphy ('Bone scan')**

Bone scintigraphy involves the administration of 99m Tc methylene diphosphonate (Tc-MDP), which is taken up by osteoblasts at sites of increased bone turnover, which may be due to tumour, trauma, infection, or degenerative disease. Increased tracer uptake is detected by a gamma camera. Spatial resolution can be further improved with single photon emission computed tomography (SPECT) imaging.

Bone scintigraphy is sensitive, and has been the standard investigation to assess the presence and extent of metastatic bone disease. The classic appearance of widespread bony malignancy is the 'super-scan', where all tracer is taken up in bone and there is no renal excretion (Figure 5.7).

However, bone scintigraphy does not have the specificity of diagnosis associated with plain film radiography, i.e. it is unable to discriminate as reliably as plain film radiography between bone metastases and alternative pathologies such as Paget's disease. (In circumstances where there is clinical doubt, a combination of isotope bone scan and plain radiography is frequently used.)

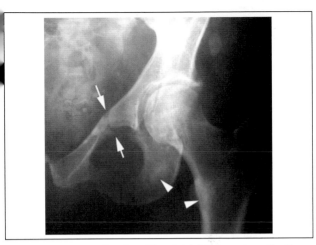

Figure 5.4 Plain radiograph performed for pain in left hip in a patient with a history of metastatic breast cancer. There is an undisplaced pathological fracture of the left superior pubic ramus in an area of sclerotic bones (arrows). Elsewhere there are other areas of bony sclerosis (arrow heads).

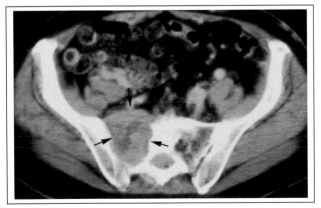

Figure 5.5 CT scan of patient with renal cell carcinoma and pain in the right leg. The plain radiograph was normal, but a CT scan demonstrates a soft tissue density destroying the sacrum to the right of the midline, and extending up to the sacro-iliac joint. A limited soft tissue mass is associated with the lesion (arrows).

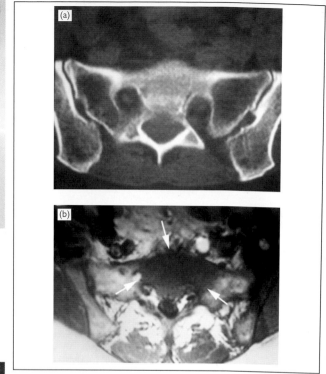

Figure 5.6 (a) CT scan at level of upper sacrum reconstructed on bony windows is within normal limits. (b) MRI undertaken 3 days later as a result of persistent pain shows extensive marrow infiltration by metastatic melanoma (arrows).

5.5 **Magnetic resonance imaging (MRI)**

MRI uses a combination of high strength magnetic fields with radio frequency pulses. Different contrast properties result from using sequences that vary the time between pulses, and anatomical localization is achieved by using magnetic gradients. These sequences allow for visualization of different structures depending on their water content. With MRI's multiplanar capability, the imaging plane can be optimized for the anatomic area being studied.

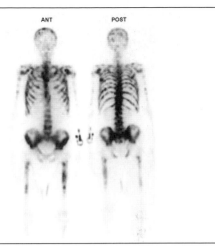

Figure 5.7 Anterior and posterior views of isotope bone scan following administration of Tc-MDP. There is increased uptake in pelvis, spine, ribs, skull and long bones. The kidneys are not demonstrated, which indicates that all isotope has been taken up by metastatic bony tumour. This appearance is known as a 'superscan'.

Ionizing radiation is not involved, and therefore it is safe to use on young patients. However, not everyone is suitable for MRI, with contraindications including patients with pacemakers and certain prostheses and surgical clips. Some patients find the procedure claustrophobic, although newer sequences allow for very rapid scans. Indeed, some patients will require sedation, or even general anaesthesia, in order to undertake a scan.

The advantage of MRI over both conventional radiography and CT is its ability to detect disease before there is any cortical destruction, i.e. its ability to detect bone marrow involvement. Bone marrow contains fat, which produces either an intermediate or high signal on T1-weighted images: the signal returned from fatty marrow contrasts well with tumour on these types of image (Figure 5.8).

However, interpretation of bone marrow signal is subjective, and requires a degree of experience. Some scans are equivocal, and follow-up imaging or further investigation may be necessary. On occasions, bone marrow involvement by tumour is complete and uniform. Under these circumstances, comparison of the marrow signal with adjacent intervertebral discs may be the only clue to extensive bony metastatic disease (Figure 5.9).

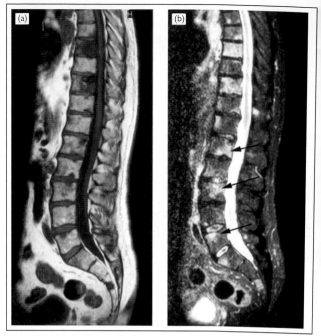

Figure 5.8 (a) Sagittal T1-weighted images of the lower thoracic and lumbar spine. There are multiple areas of low signal suggestive of metastatic disease (e.g. T8, T10, L1). (b) Short tau inversion recovery (STIR) image in sagittal plane confirms abnormal signal typical of metastatic disease. The STIR sequence is more sensitive and reveals abnormality, which is more convincing and more extensive in some vertebrae such as L1, L3 and L5 (arrows).

T1-weighted scans form the mainstay of imaging for skeletal metastases. The short tau inversion recovery sequence (STIR) is sensitive to increased water content in the marrow, and is used to clarify the situation when the T1 sequences are equivocal (Figure 5.8). Some authors have proposed a whole body STIR imaging technique. However, this has not become a mainstream investigation, and, in our experience, lacks sensitivity in the skull and extremities.

The isotope bone scan remains a sound initial investigation, as it is possible to image the entire skeleton. However, if there remains a strong clinical suspicion of bony metastatic disease, and particularly if

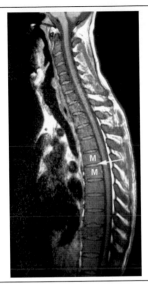

Figure 5.9 T1-weighted sagittal images of cervical and thoracic spine show diffuse homogeneous signal throughout the vertebral marrow. However, the intervertebral discs (arrow) return a higher, white signal compared with the adjacent marrow (M). This is the reversal of the normally observed signal on this sequence, and indicates that the bone marrow is entirely replaced by tumour (metastatic rhabdomyo-sarcoma).

there is focal pain, MRI is a more sensitive investigation. Thus, MRI will detect metastases in ~7% patients that have a normal isotope bone scan (Jones *et al.*, 1990).

5.6 **Positron emission tomography (PET)**

PET is a recent advance in functional imaging, using the principle of positron annihilation producing two 511 KeV gamma rays emitted at 180°, and then using coincidence detection. This gives the capability of more precise anatomical localization.

Fluorine-18 (^{18}F) is the most commonly used positron emitting tracer: it is produced in a cyclotron, but has the disadvantages of a high production cost and a short half-life of 110 min. [18]F has similar properties to Tc-MDP, although it has been suggested that PET with ^{18}F has greater sensitivity than a bone scan with Tc-MDP (at least in patients with bone metastases from breast cancer) (Schirrmeister *et al.*, 1999).

45

^{18}F fluorodeoxyglucose (FDG) combines ^{18}F with an analogue of glucose. FDG uptake reflects intracellular metabolic activity, and is therefore taken up by tissues with increased metabolic rate such as tumours. FDG PET has been shown to have increased sensitivity and specificity when compared with Tc-MDP bone scan (Bury et al., 1998; Ohta et al., 2001), and increased sensitivity when compared with MRI (Daldrup-Link et al., 2001).

Recent advances have meant that the PET image can be combined with a CT image, giving both functional and anatomical information. (PET-CT is not readily available at present.)

5.7 **Imaging in vertebral fractures**

Vertebral collapse may have a malignant cause, or a benign cause such as osteoporosis trauma, Paget's disease, and haemangioma. Furthermore, patients with a diagnosis of cancer may have both benign and malignant causes of vertebral collapse. For example, in autopsy studies of patients with known malignancy up to 30% of compression fractures are found to be benign in origin (Fornasier and Czitrom, 1978).

It is often not possible to distinguish the cause of vertebral collapse from plain radiographs. Nevertheless, the degree of collapse is generally greater in malignant disease, and there is often so-called vertebra plana (i.e. the vertebral body is crushed into a thin plate). The site of fracture can help to differentiate, with upper thoracic vertebral compression fractures more likely to be malignant than benign in nature. In addition, irregular end plates, posterior element involvement, and multiple vertebral collapses are seen more commonly in malignant disease. It should be noted that osteopenia alone cannot distinguish benign from malignant causes.

In many cases further imaging is required. CT, MRI and nuclear medicine can all be used. Laredo et al. (1995) described the CT findings in benign and malignant vertebral compression fractures, and these findings have been supported by other authors (Kubota et al., 2005) (Table 5.1).

MRI can also be very instructive in determining the cause of vertebral collapse. Uetani et al. (2004) reviewed the literature, and proposed certain criteria for discriminating between benign and malignant collapse (Table 5.2).

A variety of MRI protocols has been described, including post-intravenous gadolinium contrast images that show enhancement in metastatic collapse (Shih et al., 1999). However, the most persuasive feature for diagnosis of metastatic vertebral collapse is the detection

Table 5.1 CT features of benign and malignant vertebral collapse

Features suggesting benign cause for vertebral collapse on CT

Cortical fractures of the body without cortical bone loss

Retropulsion of bone fragments into the spinal canal

Fracture lines within cancellous bone

Intravertebral vacuum phenomenon

Thin diffuse paraspinal soft tissue mass

Features suggesting malignant cause for vertebral collapse on CT

Destruction of cancellous bone

Destruction of pedicles

Destruction of the anterolateral or posterior cortical bone

Focal paraspinal soft tissue mass or epidural mass

Table 5.2 MRI features of benign and malignant vertebral collapse

MRI features suggesting benign cause for vertebral collapse

- Band-like area of low signal intensity adjacent to depressed endplate
- Preservation of signal intensity of the vertebra

MRI features suggesting malignant cause for vertebral collapse

- Homogeneous and diffuse abnormal signal intensity
- Posterior convexity
- Involvement of the pedicles
- Paraspinal or epidural soft tissue mass
- Contrast enhancement greater than normal bone marrow

of the typical appearance of metastatic deposits in other vertebrae. The high sensitivity of MRI, and the ability to cover the whole spine, makes it a very useful test in this clinical setting (Figure 5.10).

Nuclear medicine has a limited role in differentiating benign from malignant vertebral collapse. An acute vertebral fracture of any cause will show increased uptake on the MDP bone scan, and so a diagnosis of metastatic disease can only be made by observing a multiplicity of lesions. Normalization of uptake will occur in benign vertebral fractures, but this may take up to 2 years to happen (Matin, 1979).

Zhuang et al. (2003) have studied FDG-PET in the context of bony fracture and found that increased uptake is also present in the acute phase, but normalizes more quickly than the MDP scan. Thus, FDG uptake will return to normal within 3 months of a traumatic fracture, although uptake will be more persistent in cases of infection or malignancy.

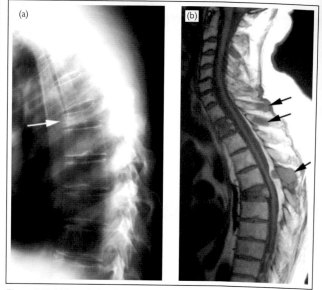

Figure 5.10 (a) Lateral plain film of thoracic spine shows collapse of a mid-thoracic vertebra (arrow). (b) Sagittal T1-weighted MRI confirms vertebral collapse at T6, and a further lesion at T2. The posterior elements of T5 are expanded by tumour and there are further areas of low signal in the posterior elements of T1 and T2 (arrows). The finding of expansion of bone, involvement of the posterior elements and multiplicity of lesions indicate that the vertebral collapse is of malignant aetiology (multiple myeloma).

5.8 **Imaging in multiple myeloma**

Myeloma is characterised by multiple lytic bone lesions. The degree of bone involvement influences management and, therefore, the extent of the disease needs to be adequately established.

For many years the skeletal survey with plain radiographs has been the mainstay of initial assessment and subsequent follow-up. This includes radiographs of the skull, the whole spine, the chest, the pelvis, both humeri and both femurs. Additional views are sometimes added if there is an area of clinical concern. However, the sensitivity of the radiographs is low: 50% of the bone must be destroyed before a lesion is visible on a radiograph (Edelstyn et al., 1967).

MDP bone scan has been shown to be of limited use as the lesions cause very little osteoblastic activity. Radiopharmaceuticals such as gallium 67, thallium 201 chloride and technetium-99m sestamibi have been more successful at identifying sites of disease. Of these Tc-99m sestamibi is the most widely used, although its use has been somewhat superseded by MRI.

MRI is being used more often in myeloma. The most common site of disease is the lower thoracic and lumbar spine, and MRI of the spine has been shown to be more sensitive than plain films and isotope bone scan (and has the advantage of assessing for spinal canal invasion and cord suppression) (Ludwig *et al.*, 1987). However, up to 20% of patients with established myeloma have normal MRI examinations despite diffuse bone marrow involvement (Lecouvet *et al.*, 1999). There has been some recent interest in rapid whole body MRI techniques in myeloma, with increased lesion detection claimed when compared to plain radiographs and CT scanning (van de Berg *et al.*, 1996; Arcuti *et al.*, 2005; Buhmann *et al.*, 2005).

FDG-PET imaging can detect myelomatous deposits as there is increased metabolic activity within lesions. PET scans have the advantage of assessing the whole body, and have been shown to be more sensitive than plain radiographs for lesion detection (Schirrmeister *et al.*, 2002). Furthermore, PET scans can identify extramedullary lesions. There has been no direct comparison between PET and MRI imaging in myeloma, although there are studies in progress. At present, FDG-PET imaging remains a useful adjunct to other imaging modalities.

5.9 **Conclusion**

The imaging of bone pain due to suspected malignancy requires a multi-modal approach. In almost all cases a plain radiograph should be the first investigation as this is widely available, easy to perform and easily repeatable. Following this, the investigation pathway should be guided by the clinical situation, and in the current climate of evolving imaging techniques it is a good idea to consult specialists in diagnostic imaging prior to subjecting the patient to the full weight of imaging technology.

References

Arcuti, P., Fumagalli, I., Zacchino, M., *et al.* (2005). Whole body MRI for detecting multiple myeloma bone marrow infiltration: correlation to contrast-enhanced MRI and roentgen ray radiography. *Radiology*, **237** (Suppl. Dec.), 449.

Buhmann, S., Schoenberg, S., Becker, C., Reiser, M., and Baur-Melnyk, A. (2005). Imaging diagnostics in patients with multiple myeloma: whole body MDCT versus whole body MRI. *Radiology*, **237** (Suppl. Dec.), 449.

Bury, T., Barreto, A., Daenen, F., Barthelemy, N., Ghaye, B., and Rigo, P. (1998). Fluorine-18 deoxyglucose positron emission tomography for the detection of bone metastases in patients with non-small cell lung cancer. *Eur. J. Nucl. Med.*, **25**, 1244–7.

Daldrup-Link, H.E., Franzius, C., Link, T.M. *et al.* (2001). Whole-body MR imaging for detection of bone metastases in children and young adults: comparison with skeletal scintigraphy and FDG PET. *Am. J. Roentgenol.*, **177**, 229–36.

Edelstyn, G.A., Gillespie, P.J., and Grebbell, F.S. (1967). The radiological demonstration of osseous metastases. Experimental observations. *Clin. Radiol.*, **18**, 158–62.

Fornasier, V.L., and Czitrom, A.A. (1978). Collapsed vertebrae: a review of 659 autopsies. *Clin. Orthop. Related Res.*, **131**, 261–5.

Jones, A.L., Williams, M.P., Powles, T.J. *et al.* (1990). Magnetic resonance imaging in the detection of skeletal metastases in patients with breast cancer. *Br. J. Cancer*, **62**, 296–8.

Kubota, T., Yamada, K., Ito, H., Kizu, O., and Nishimura, T. (2005). High-resolution imaging of the spine using multidetector-row computed tomography: differentiation between benign and malignant vertebral compression fractures. *J. Comput. Assist. Tomogr.*, **29**, 712–9.

Laredo, J.D., Lakhdari, K., Bellaïche, L., Hamze, B., Janklewicz, P., and Tubiana, J.M. (1995). Acute vertebral collapse: CT findings in benign and malignant nontraumatic cases. *Radiology*, **194**, 41–8.

Lecouvet, F.E., Malghem, J., Michaux, L. *et al.* (1999). Skeletal survey in advanced multiple myeloma: radiographic versus MR imaging survey. *Br. J. Haematol.*, **106**, 35–9.

Ludwig, H., Fruhwald, F., Tscholakoff, D., Rasoul, S., Neuhold, A., and Fritz, E. (1987). Magnetic resonance imaging of the spine in multiple myeloma. *Lancet*, **2**, 364–6.

Matin, P. (1979). The appearance of bone scans following fractures, including immediate and long-term studies. *J. Nucl. Med.*, **20**, 1227–31.

Ohta, M., Tokuda, Y., Suzuki, Y. *et al.* (2001). Whole body PET for the evaluation of bony metastases in patients with breast cancer: comparison with 99Tcm-MDP bone scintigraphy. *Nucl. Med. Commun.*, **22**, 875–9.

Schirrmeister, H., Guhlmann, A., Kotzerke, J. *et al.* (1999). Early detection and accurate description of extent of metastatic bone disease in breast cancer with fluoride ion and positron emission tomography. *J. Clin. Oncol.*, **17**, 2381–9.

Schirrmeister, H., Bommer, M., Buck, A.K. *et al.* (2002). Initial results in the assessment of multiple myeloma using 18F-FDG PET. *Eur. J. Nucl. Med. Mol. Imag.*, **29**, 361–6.

Shih, T.T., Huang, K.M., and Li, Y.W. (1999). Solitary vertebral collapse: distinction between benign and malignant causes using MR patterns. *J. Magn. Reson. Imag.*, **9**, 635–42.

Uetani, M., Hashmi, R., and Hayashi, K. (2004). Malignant and benign compression fractures: differentiation and diagnostic pitfalls on MRI. *Clin. Radiol.*, **59**, 124–31.

Van de Berg, B.C., Lecouvet, F.E., Michaux, L. *et al.* (1996). Stage 1 multiple myeloma: value of MR imaging of the bone marrow in the determination of prognosis. *Radiology*, **201**, 243–6.

Zhuang, H., Sam, J.W., Chacko, T.K. *et al.* (2003). Rapid normalization of osseous FDG uptake following traumatic or surgical fractures. *Eur. J. Nucl. Med. Mol. Imag.*, **30**, 1096–103.

Chapter 6

Conventional analgesics for bone pain

John Zeppetella

6.1 Introduction

Patients with cancer-induced bone pain (CIBP) often report that their pain varies during the course of the day. In general, two types of pain pattern can be identified: a continuous pain ('background pain'); and a transitory exacerbation of pain ('breakthrough pain'). This chapter will review the evidence for the effectiveness of conventional analgesics in the management of both background and breakthrough CIBP (i.e. non-opioid analgesics, opioid analgesics). It should be noted that some patients with CIBP may require additional forms of pharmacological intervention to deal with associated muscle spasm (e.g. benzodiazepines), or nerve impingement (e.g. corticosteroids).

6.2 Background pain

6.2.1 General principles

Oral pharmacological management is usually the first line in the treatment of bone pain in patients with cancer. Management does not generally differ from other types of cancer pain, and uses the World Health Organization (WHO, 1996) analgesic guidelines. Presented in the form of a three-step ladder, the WHO recommends a non-opioid (e.g. paracetamol, non-steroidal anti-inflammatory drug) for mild pain at step 1, an 'opioid for mild to moderate pain' (e.g. codeine, dihydrocodeine) at step 2, and an 'opioid for moderate to severe pain' (e.g. morphine, oxycodone) at step 3; analgesia is delivered according to the severity of the pain and not the severity of the disease (see Figure 4.2).

It has been argued that it would be difficult to know whether the WHO ladder has really improved the management of cancer pain as none of the published studies is a randomized controlled trial, and some are retrospective, some have variable/short follow-up and some have large numbers of withdrawals (Jadad and Browman, 1995). Others have taken a more pragmatic view that the published studies include almost 4000 patients, that the results were consistent across different clinical settings and countries, that there is a considerable body of additional supporting (anecdotal) evidence, and that it would be impossible to conduct a randomized controlled trial now that the WHO method has become a world standard (Hanks and Hawkins, 2000).

The following sections will examine the evidence for conventional analgesics (i.e. non-opioid analgesics, opioid analgesics) in the management of cancer-related pain, and specifically in the management of CIBP.

6.2.2 **Non-opioid analgesics**

Paracetamol (acetaminophen)

Paracetamol is one of the most commonly used analgesics, and is widely available without prescription throughout the world. It has antipyretic and analgesic actions, but despite being available for over 100 years the mechanism of action of paracetamol remains unclear. It has been suggested that paracetamol selectively inhibits the enzyme COX-3, a spliced variant of COX-1, in the brain and spinal cord, which could explain the effectiveness of paracetamol in reducing fever and relieving pain without having the unwanted gastrointestinal adverse effects typical of non-steroidal anti-inflammatory drugs. Others have argued that this action is unlikely to be clinically relevant, and that the analgesic effect of paracetamol is due to activation of descending serotonergic pathways within the central nervous system (Graham and Scott, 2005).

The evidence for the analgesic efficacy of paracetamol is primarily in acute post-operative pain. A systematic review of 74 trials (6372 participants) showed that paracetamol is an effective analgesic, with a low incidence of adverse effects, in this setting (Moore et al., 2000). A recent systematic review of non-opioids in the management of cancer pain included paracetamol within its search terms, but did not analyse paracetamol separately due to insufficient data (McNichol et al., 2004). The review identified two studies involving paracetamol, neither of which was concerned with CIBP. Studies examining a possible additive analgesic effect of paracetamol on opioid therapy in cancer patients (including patients with CIBP) have produced conflicting results [Axelsson and Borup, 2003; Stockler et al., 2004].

In summary, therefore, there is little evidence to support the role of paracetamol in the management of CIBP.

Non-steroidal anti-inflammatory drugs (NSAIDs)

NSAIDs are one of the most widely prescribed drugs with >30 million people worldwide using prescription NSAIDs on a daily basis (Singh, 2000). NSAIDs reduce the biosynthesis of prostaglandins by inhibiting cyclo-oxygenase (COX), and the cascade of inflammatory events that cause, amplify, or maintain nociception. Other possible mechanisms of action include an effect on the cell membranes of neutrophils to inhibit the release of inflammatory mediators, a central effect on pain perception, and an effect on N-methyl-d-aspartate (NMDA) receptors to reduce NMDA-mediated hyperalgesia (Jenkins and Bruera, 1999).

NSAIDs are recommended at step 1 of the analgesic ladder, although they can also be used in combination with opioids at steps 2/3 of the analgesic ladder. Many preparations are available, differing in drug, dose, formulation, adverse effects, drug interactions and cost. Studies suggest that there is little difference in the effectiveness of NSAIDs among populations (Eisenberg et al., 1994; McNichol et al., 2004), but effectiveness and adverse effects vary markedly from patient to patient.

A systematic review of randomized controlled clinical trials of NSAIDs for cancer pain was published in 2004 (McNichol et al., 2004). It included 42 trials involving 3084 patients. The review concluded that NSAIDs were effective for the short term treatment of cancer pain, and that there was no clear evidence to support a superior efficacy or safety of one NSAID over another. It included 14 trials involving patients with bone metastases, although the authors were unable to conclude from the data presented whether NSAIDs have a specific role in CIBP.

The results of this systematic review were in keeping with the results of an earlier systematic review of the literature on NSAIDs for cancer pain (Eisenberg et al., 1994), and a concurrent evidence-based review of the literature on the generic treatment of cancer pain (Carr et al., 2004). It should be noted that many of the trials included in these reviews are single-dose studies, and few of the trials evaluate the efficacy or safety of NSAIDs beyond a few days of treatment.

In summary, therefore, there is a lack of evidence for a specific role for NSAIDs in the management of CIBP.

6.2.2 Opioid analgesics

According to the WHO analgesic ladder, opioids are utilized at both step 2 ('opioids for mild to moderate pain') and step 3 ('opioids for moderate to severe pain') (WHO, 1996). Despite studies reporting that use of the WHO ladder can result in good analgesia in most patients with cancer pain (Hanks and Hawkins, 2000), there are instances where patients with CIBP are either not prescribed opioids, or still have uncontrolled pain despite step 3 opioids (Yau et al., 2004).

The systematic reviews on NSAIDs for cancer pain included comparative studies with opioids and combinations of NSAIDs and opioids. In the earlier review, single or multiple doses of step 2 opioids did not produce greater analgesia than NSAIDs alone, and in single doses step 2 opioids produced more adverse effects than NSAIDs, although there was an equal prevalence following multiple doses (Eisenberg et al., 1994). (These results led the authors to question the value of step 2 of the WHO analgesic ladder.) The later review also concluded that combinations of NSAIDs and opioid (step 2 and step 3) either showed no difference, or at best a slight difference, compared to each drug given separately (McNichol et al., 2004). In both reviews there was no specific evidence regarding opioids and CIBP.

The evidence-based review of the literature on the generic treatment of cancer pain identified 23 randomized controlled trials involving the use of opioid analgesics (1870 patients in total) (Carr et al., 2004). The authors concluded that opioids administered via various routes can relieve moderate to severe cancer pain. Unfortunately, the reporting of included studies did not allow for a separate analysis of CIBP.

It is generally accepted that opioids are best administered regularly 'around-the-clock' (Hanks et al., 2001). However, a study of 137 oncology outpatients with pain from bone metastases appeared to show that patients using opioids on an 'as-required basis' had similar pain relief compared to patients taking opioids around-the-clock, despite using on average lower daily doses of opioid (Miaskowski et al., 2002).

The step 3 opioids used most commonly in palliative care are morphine, oxycodone, fentanyl, hydromorphone, and methadone; the results of Cochrane systematic reviews for each of these opioids are summarized below.

Morphine

Morphine is a pure opioid agonist with particular affinity for the mu receptor. Morphine is well absorbed by all routes of administration; when given orally it has a highly variable oral bioavailability (mean 33%; range 16–68%) resulting in wide dosing requirements and a broad spectrum of response. Morphine is recommended as the opioid of first choice for the management of moderate to severe cancer pain by the European Association for Palliative Care (EAPC) (Hanks et al., 2001).

A systematic review of oral morphine for cancer pain identified 45 randomized controlled trials (3061 patients), and included studies comparing different preparations, formulations, administration routes, strengths, and dose frequencies; studies comparing morphine to other opioids and non-opioids were also included (Wiffen et al., 2003). The review concluded that morphine is an effective analgesic. No distinction was made in the review between CIBP and non-CIBP.

Oxycodone

Oxycodone is a semi-synthetic thebaine derivative that is suitable for oral administration due to its high bioavailability (60%); it may also be given intramuscularly, intravenously, subcutaneously, and rectally. In 1996 it was launched in the UK as an alternative to oral morphine, and has been recommended as such by the EAPC (Hanks et al., 2001).

Two recent reviews identified six randomized controlled trials where oxycodone was used for cancer pain (Reid et al., 2002; Kalso, 2005). One review reported detailed analysis of four studies (181 patients), and concluded that oxycodone has similar efficacy, and tolerability, to morphine (Reid et al., 2002); no data were available relating to CIBP (Andrew Davies, personal communication).

Fentanyl

Fentanyl is a synthetic opioid related to the phenylpiperidines. It is primarily a mu agonist and is estimated to be 100 times more potent than morphine. Fentanyl was initially introduced into clinical practice as an intravenous preparation for anaesthesia and peri-operative analgesia, but its low molecular weight and high lipid solubility led to the subsequent development of a transdermal therapeutic system.

A review of randomized controlled trials where fentanyl was used for chronic pain identified eight studies, four of which were in a cancer pain setting (427 patients in total) (Ribeiro and Zeppetella, 2006). Fentanyl was shown to be as effective an analgesic as morphine in cancer pain, and in some cases had fewer adverse effects. Although patients' primary diagnoses were usually described in the included studies, there were no specific references to CIBP.

Hydromorphone

Hydromorphone is an analogue of morphine with similar pharmacokinetic and pharmacodynamic properties. It was first introduced in the UK in 1997, as an alternative to morphine in the management of cancer pain. However, it had been used to treat cancer pain in other countries for many years.

A systematic review of randomized controlled trials of hydromorphone identified 43 studies, 11 of which involved cancer pain (645 participants in total) (Quigley, 2002). The results suggest that hydromorphone is of similar efficacy to morphine, and has a similar adverse effect profile; there was no specific analysis of CIBP.

Methadone

Methadone is a synthetic opioid that is primarily a mu agonist, although it also has δ-opioid receptor agonist properties, and is a pre-synaptic blocker of serotonin re-uptake. Methadone is a highly lipophilic molecule that is suitable for a variety of administration routes; oral bioavailability of methadone is ~80%. However, methadone's unpredictable (long) half-life can result in accumulation, and make its use very complicated in some patients.

A systematic review of randomized controlled trials in cancer pain identified eight trials, which involved 356 patients (Nicholson, 2004). The review concluded that methadone has a similar efficacy to morphine, and a comparable side-effect profile. Two of the studies described pain types (including bone pain), although no relationship between efficacy and type of pain was reported.

In summary, there are a number of published open studies reporting the efficacy of both step 2 and step 3 opioids for CIBP, although as discussed above evidence from randomized controlled trials is lacking. In recent years there has been increasing use of the practices of opioid switching and combining different opioids; in both cases the aim is to improve pain control and reduce adverse effects. At present there are no controlled studies focusing on these practices for the management of CIBP.

6.3 Breakthrough pain

Breakthrough pain is an intermittent, transient exacerbation of pain that occurs spontaneously ('spontaneous pain'), or in relation to a predictable or unpredictable trigger ('incident pain'), usually in spite of ongoing analgesic therapy. It is a heterogeneous phenomenon, although it is typically of fast onset, short duration, and feels much like background pain except that it may be more severe.

Breakthrough pain is often difficult to manage. Thus, despite implementation of guidelines, patients continue to have inadequate pain control, and often express dissatisfaction with their treatment. Incident breakthrough pain, triggered by movement, can be particularly difficult to control (Banning et al., 1991). (This type of breakthrough pain is invariably related to the presence of underlying bone metastases.)

Three principles have been proposed for the management of breakthrough pain (Portenoy, 1997):

1. Implementation of primary therapies for the underlying aetiology of the pain.
2. Optimizing around-the-clock medication.
3. Specific pharmacological or non-pharmacological interventions for the breakthrough pain.

It has been suggested that increasing around-the-clock medication may prevent or limit breakthrough pain associated with CIBP (Mercadante et al., 2004a). Thus, 25 patients admitted to a palliative care unit with incident breakthrough pain were titrated with intravenous morphine to background pain relief. The morphine dose was then increased further until patients began to experience adverse effects, at which point the increase was either stopped, or the morphine dose reduced. Patients remained as inpatients for an average of 5 days, and the breakthrough pain intensity fell from an average of 9.2 before titration to 4.6 at the time of discharge. Most patients tolerated the higher doses of morphine.

The commonest method of managing breakthrough pain is by the use of so-called rescue medication ('breakthrough medication'). Ideally, rescue medication should have an onset/duration of action appropriate for the pain, should have a potency of effect appropriate for the pain, and be easily administered. Rescue medication should be offered soon after the pain has started in cases of unpredictable pain, and before the pain has started in cases of predictable pain.

Non-opioids such as NSAIDs could have a role in the management of breakthrough pain as their mode of action suggests that they would be efficacious. However, with an onset of action of ~30 min, a relatively long duration of action, and dose-limiting adverse effects, they are not ideally suited to the management of breakthrough pain. Furthermore, there are no studies to suggest that they are effective in this clinical scenario.

Opioids are commonly used as rescue medication. Morphine, hydromorphone and oxycodone are the most common oral opioids used, and a fixed proportion of the daily dose is usually advised (e.g. the 4 hourly dose equivalent) (Hanks et al., 2001). One study formally assessed the use of a fixed dose of rescue medication (Mercadante et al., 2004b): 48 patients using oral morphine for background cancer pain, and admitted to a palliative care unit, were treated with intravenous morphine equivalent to one-fifth of the around-the-clock dose for management of their breakthrough pain. A total of 172 episodes of pain were assessed, and most patients had a 33% reduction of their pain within 18 min. Although most patients had somatic cancer pain, there was no specific reference to CIBP. It should be noted that the effects of most oral opioids last longer than the episode of incident breakthrough pain, and so patients may experience adverse effects after the pain has subsided.

A systematic review on the use of opioids for breakthrough pain identified four studies, each concerned with the application of oral transmucosal fentanyl citrate (Zeppetella and Ribeiro, 2006). Oral transmucosal fentanyl citrate (OTFC) is a sweetened lozenge containing fentanyl on a stick, specifically developed for the management of breakthrough pain (Figure 6.1). The lozenge is rubbed against the inside of the cheek, and the fentanyl diffuses into the circulation. The fast onset of OTFC (comparable to intravenous morphine), and the rapid redistribution, renders it ideally suited to the management of breakthrough pain.

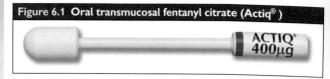

Figure 6.1 Oral transmucosal fentanyl citrate (Actiq®)

ACTIQ®
400µg

The aforementioned studies confirmed the efficacy of this delivery system for the management of breakthrough pain (Christie *et al.*, 1998; Farrar *et al.*, 1998; Portenoy *et al.*, 1999; Coluzzi *et al.*, 2001), and one demonstrated that OTFC was superior to morphine in the management of breakthrough pain (Coluzzi *et al.*, 2001). However, all of the studies failed to demonstrate a relationship between the effective dose of OTFC and the effective dose of around-the-clock medication, and as a result the optimum dose is determined by titration. Most of 393 patients in the studies had nociceptive pain, the majority of which were somatic in type. However, although one study did describe the number of patients with CIBP (Christie *et al.*, 1998), none of the studies distinguished between CIBP and non-CIBP in their analyses.

In summary, therefore, the strongest evidence is for OTFC, which has been specifically developed for the management of breakthrough pain. There is, however, no published evidence for a specific role of OTFC in CIBP.

6.4 **Conclusion**

In clinical practice the management of CIBP generally follows the same principles as the management of other types of (somatic) nociceptive pain. Although there is evidence in the literature which supports the role of both non-opioids and opioids in the management of both background and breakthrough cancer pain, the heterogeneity of study designs makes it difficult to find evidence specifically supporting a role for these drugs in CIBP.

References

Axelsson, B., and Borup, S. (2003). Is there an additive analgesic effect of paracetamol at step 3? A double-blind randomized controlled study. *Palliative Medicine*, **17**, 724–5.

Banning, A., Sjogren, P., and Henriksen, H. (1991). Treatment outcome in a multidisciplinary cancer pain clinic. *Pain*, **47**, 129–34.

Carr, D.B., Goudas, L.C., Balk, E.M., Bloch, R., Ioannidis, J.P., and Lau, J. (2004). Evidence report on the treatment of pain in cancer patients. *J. Nat. Cancer Inst.*, *Monographs* (**32**), 23–31.

Christie, J.M., Simmonds, M., Patt, R. et al. (1998). Dose-titration, multicenter study of oral transmucosal fentanyl citrate for the treatment of breakthrough pain in cancer patients using transdermal fentanyl for persistent pain. *J. Clin. Oncol.*, **16**, 3238–45.

Coluzzi, P.H., Schwartzberg, L., Conroy Jr, J.D. et al. (2001). Breakthrough cancer pain: a randomized trial comparing oral transmucosal fentanyl citrate (OTFC) and morphine sulfate immediate release (MSIR). *Pain*, **91**, 123–30.

Eisenberg, E., Berkey, C.S., Carr, D.B., Mosteller, F., and Chalmers, T.C. (1994). Efficacy and safety of nonsteroidal antiinflammatory drugs for cancer pain: a meta-analysis. *J. Clin. Oncology*, **12**, 2756–65.

Farrar, J.T., Cleary, J., Rauck, R., Busch, M., and Nordbrock, F. (1998). Oral transmucosal fentanyl citrate: randomized, double-blinded, placebo-controlled trial for treatment of breakthrough pain in cancer patients. *J. Nat. Cancer Inst.*, **90**, 611–6.

Graham, G.G., and Scott, K.F. (2005). Mechanism of action of paracetamol. *Am. J. Therapeut.*, **12**, 46–55.

Hanks, G.W., and Hawkins, C. (2000). Agreeing a gold standard in the management of cancer pain: the role of opioids. In: Hillier, R., Finlay, I., Welsh, J., and Miles, A., (ed.) The effective management of cancer pain, pp. 57–77. Aesculapius Medical Press, London.

Hanks, G.W., de Conno, F., Cherny, N. et al. (2001). Morphine and alternative opioids in cancer pain: the EAPC recommendations. *Br. J. Cancer*, **84**, 587–93.

Jadad, A.R., and Browman, G.P. (1995). The WHO analgesic ladder for cancer pain management. Stepping up the quality of its evaluation. *JAMA*, **274**, 1870–3.

Jenkins, C.A., and Bruera, E. (1999). Nonsteroidal anti-inflammatory drugs as adjuvant analgesics in cancer patients. *Palliat. Med.*, **13**, 183–96.

Kalso, E. (2005). Oxycodone. *J. Pain Sympt. Management*, **29** (5 Suppl.), S47–56.

McNicol, E., Strassels, S., Goudas, L., Lau, J., and Carr, D. (2004). Nonsteroidal anti-inflammatory drugs, alone or combined with opioids, for cancer pain: a systematic review. *J. Clin. Oncol.*, **22**, 1975–92.

Mercadante, S., Villari, P., Ferrera, P., and Casuccio, A. (2004a). Optimization of opioid therapy for preventing incident pain associated with bone metastases. *J. Pain Sympt. Management*, **28**, 505–10.

Mercadante, S., Villari, P., Ferrera, P., Bianchi, M., and Casuccio, A. (2004b). Safety and effectiveness of intravenous morphine for episodic (breakthrough) pain using a fixed ratio with the oral daily morphine dose. *J. Pain Sympt. Management*, **27**, 352–9.

Miaskowski, C., Mack, K.A., Dodd, M. et al. (2002). Oncology patients with pain from bone metastases require more than around-the-clock dosing of analgesia to achieve adequate pain control. *J. Pain*, **3**, 12–20.

Moore, A., Collins, S., Carroll, D., McQuay, H., and Edwards, J. (2000). Single dose paracetamol (acetaminophen), with and without codeine, for postoperative pain. Cochrane Database *Syst. Rev.*, (2), CD001547.

Nicholson, A.B. (2004). Methadone for cancer pain. *Cochrane Database Syst. Rev.*, (2), CD003971.

Portenoy, R.K. (1997). Treatment of temporal variations in chronic cancer pain. *Semin. Oncol.*, **5**, S16–7-12.

Portenoy, R.K., Payne, R., Coluzzi, P. *et al.* (1999). Oral transmucosal fentanyl citrate (OTFC) for the treatment of breakthrough pain in cancer patients: a controlled dose titration study. *Pain*, **79**, 303–12.

Quigley, C. (2002). Hydromorphone for acute and chronic pain. *Cochrane Database Syst. Rev.*, (1), CD003447.

Reid, C.M., Davies, A.N., Hanks, G.W. Oxycodone for cancer-related pain. *Cochrane Database Syst. Rev.* (in press).

Ribeiro, M.D., Zeppetella, G. Fentanyl for chronic pain. *Cochrane Database Syst. Rev.* (in press).

Singh, G. (2000). Gastrointestinal complications of prescription and over-the-counter nonsteroidal anti-inflammatory drugs: a view from the ARAMIS database. Arthritis Rheumatism, and Aging Medical Information System. *Am. J. Therapeut.*, **7**, 115–21.

Stockler, M., Vardy, J., Pillai, A., and Warr, D. (2004). Acetaminophen (paracetamol) improves pain and well-being in people with advanced cancer already receiving a strong opioid regimen: a randomized, double-blind, placebo-controlled cross-over trial. *J. Clin. Oncol.*, **22**, 3389–94.

Wiffen, P.J., Edwards, J.E., Barden, J., and McQuay, H.J. (2003). Oral morphine for cancer pain. *Cochrane Database Syst. Rev.*, (4), CD003868.

Yau, V., Chow, E., Davis, L., Holden, L., Schueller, T., and Danjoux, C. (2004). Pain management in cancer patients with bone metastases remains a challenge. *J. Pain Sympt. Management*, **27**, 1–3.

World Health Organization (1996). *Cancer pain relief* (2nd edn). WHO, Geneva.

Zeppetella, G., and Ribeiro, M.D. (2006). Opioids for the management of breakthrough (episodic) pain in cancer patients. *Cochrane Database Syst. Rev.*, (1), CD004311.

Chapter 7

Bisphosphonates for bone pain

Rebecca Wong

7.1 Introduction

In the 1960s, Fleisch and Bisaz identified substances in the blood and urine that prevented the formation and dissolution of calcium phosphate crystals, which were later characterized as pyrophosphates (Fleisch and Bisaz, 1962). Recognizing their biophysical properties, Fleisch hypothesized that pyrophosphates were an important regulator of bone mineralization and demineralization, and potentially useful in preventing or treating abnormal calcification and excessive bone destruction (Fleisch, 1987).

However, the rapid breakdown of pyrophosphates in the body was the challenge towards their clinical application. Bisphosphonates, pyrophosphate analogues created by replacing the oxygen in the pyrophosphate structure with carbon, provided the solution to this problem. Over the years, a number of different bisphosphonates have been developed, with the newer agents exhibiting increased potency as compared to the original agents.

This chapter will discuss the data on bisphosphonates in the management of cancer-related bone pain. However, bisphosphonates are also used to manage/prevent other skeletal complications of cancer (Krempien et al., 2005), and also to manage cancer-related hypercalcaemia (Stewart, 2005).

7.2 Structure of bisphosphonates

As mentioned above, bisphosphonates differ from pyrophosphates in that the phosphorus atoms are linked by a carbon atom instead of an oxygen atom. Specific bisphosphonates are further characterized by their side chains at R1 and R2 (see Figure 7.1). With side chain modifications from a simple methyl group (CH_3) to progressively longer alkyl chains, successive generations of bisphosphonates have been developed, each with increasing potency to inhibit osteoclast-mediated bone resorption.

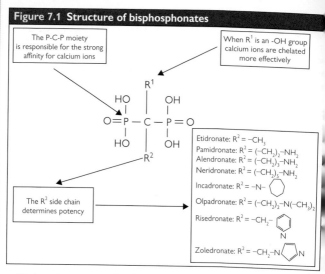

Figure 7.1 Structure of bisphosphonates

The P-C-P moiety is responsible for the strong affinity for calcium ions

When R^1 is an -OH group calcium ions are chelated more effectively

The R^2 side chain determines potency

Etidronate: R^2 = $-CH_3$
Pamidronate: R^2 = $(-CH_2)_2-NH_2$
Alendronate: R^2 = $(-CH_2)_3-NH_2$
Neridronate: R^2 = $(-CH_2)_5-NH_2$
Incadronate: R^2 = $-N-$
Olpadronate: R^2 = $(-CH_2)_2-N(-CH_3)_2$
Risedronate: R^2 = $-CH_2-$
Zoledronate: R^2 = $-CH_2-N$

Bisphosphonates can be divided into non-amino-bisphosphonates (e.g. clodronate, etidronate), and the more potent non-amino-bisphosphonates (e.g. alendronate, ibandronate, pamidronate, risedronate, zoledronate). They differ in the ability to be metabolized into analogues of ATP. Amino-bisphosphonates (after being metabolized into non-hydrolyzable ATP analogs) compete with ATP in its enzymatic function, inhibiting optimal cellular energy production within osteoclasts. In contrast, non-amino-bisphosphonates exert their effects through inhibition of the mevalonate pathway, (important in the y), which ultimately affects the synthesis of small GTPases (signalling proteins), which are in turn critical for optimal osteoclast cellular function and activity that regulate a variety of cellular processes (Santini et al., 2003).

7.3 **Action of bisphosphonates**

Bisphosphonates have a number of actions, which account for their anti-resorptive properties (Santini et al., 2003; Green, 2004). Thus, they inhibit dissolution of hydroxyapatite crystals, have an effect on osteoclasts, have an effect on osteoblasts, and also have an effect on the underlying tumour (see below). It should be noted that different bisphosphonates have a different range of activities.

Figure 7.1 is reproduced with permission from Santini, D., Vespasiani Gentilucci, U., Vincenzi, B. et al. (2003). The anti-neoplastic role of biphosphonates: from basic research to clinical evidence. Ann. Oncol. **14**: 1468–76.

Bisphosphonates can inhibit the differentiation of stem cells to osteoclasts, affect the structure and function of osteoclasts, and cause apoptosis of osteoclasts (Santini *et al.*, 2003). The latter actions rely on the bisphosphonate being taken up into the osteoclast by a process of endocytosis. Bisphosphonates also affect the interaction between ostoclasts and osteoblasts.

In addition, bisphosphonates can inhibit the growth of tumour cells, stimulate the immune system (against the tumour), and cause apoptosis of tumour cells (Santini *et al.*, 2003). The inhibition of growth is achieved by a reduction in the adhesion of tumour cells to bone, a reduction in the secretion of tumour growth factors into the bone (secondary to a reduction in bone resorption), and an inhibition of tumour angiogenesis.

7.4 **Clinical data—efficacy**

As discussed above, bisphosphonates delay the development of skeletal events, particularly in patients with breast cancer, multiple myeloma and prostate cancer (Bloomfield, 1998; Michaelson and Smith, 2005). A positive effect of delaying skeletal events is an overall reduction in pain secondary to bone resorption and its complications (e.g. pathological fracture, nerve compression).

However, bisphosphonates can also improve pain secondary to established bone lesions: many patients only respond after months of treatment, whilst other patients respond soon after treatment is initiated. The mechanism by which bisphosphonates cause long-term pain relief is likely to be due to their effect on bone resorption (and healing of the bone lesions). The mechanism by which bisphosphonates cause short term pain relief is unclear, but is likely to be related to their effect on tumour growth factors and other nociceptive agents (see Chapter 2).

A Cochrane systematic review addressing the (acute) analgesic effect of bisphosphonates was first published by Wong and Wiffen (2002). The data were subsequently updated to create a Health Technology Report for the Canadian Coordinating Center of Health Technology Assessment (Wong *et al.*, 2004). The data were further updated for the current chapter: the medical literature last searched in October 2005, and an additional six randomized trials comparing bisphosphonates with no treatment, placebo, or an active drug (Body *et al.*, 2003; Dearnaley *et al.*, 2003; Rosen *et al.*, 2003; Small *et al.*, 2003; Tripathy *et al.*, 2004; Wang *et al.*, 2004), and three trials comparing bisphosphonates with other active treatment modalities (Shucai *et al.*, 1999; Wang *et al.*, 2003; Wong *et al.*, 2003), were identified.

The following sections will describe the methodology of the review, and the results of the most recent update of the review.

Study selection

The study inclusion criteria consisted of randomized trials, patients with bone metastases, patients with or without pain at the time of enrolment, and pain as an outcome measure. In addition, one study arm had to include a bisphosphonate agent, while the other study arm could include no treatment, a placebo, a different dose of the same bisphosphonate, a different type of bisphosphonate, or a different treatment modality. Studies capturing only observer-rated pain scores were excluded from the review.

Search strategy

Multiple electronic databases were searched between the years 1966 and 2004, including MEDLINE, EMBASE, the Cochrane Library (Cochrane Controlled Trials Register), and the Oxford Pain Database. (This search was latterly supplemented with a MEDLINE search for the years 2004-2005.) A comprehensive strategy was utilized to identify randomized trials (Dickersin et al., 1994); in addition, MeSH terms and key words for bisphosphonates, bone neoplasms and pain, and the generic and trade names of bisphosphonates, were included in the search strategy.

Methods of the analysis

The key summary data extracted included the proportion of patients with pain relief, mean or median pain scores, analgesic reduction, and analgesic scores. Only data collected between weeks 0 and 12 was used in the review. In order to provide an overall assessment as to whether bisphosphonates as a class of drugs possess pain relief properties, the available data were pooled together (after establishing that the available data were homogeneous).

Secondary analyses were conducted as we were interested in whether different disease sites, and different types of bisphosphonates, possess different responses. Finally, sensitivity analyses were conducted, since several methodological assumptions were made in order to conduct the meta-analysis. The factors examined included the nature of the control arm (no treatment versus placebo), whether pain was a study entry criterion, and the methodological quality of the study (Jadad et al., 1996).

7.4.1 **Overall results**

Fifty-six trials fulfilled the selection criteria for the most recent analysis. The data support the fact that bisphosphonates provide relief of pain within 12 weeks of therapy. The odds ratio (OR) for the best response within 12 weeks was 1.87 [95% confidence interval (CI): 1.23–2.86]. The time-course of the effect was not immediate. Thus, while there was a trend towards pain relief at weeks 4 and 8, this only became statistically significant at week 12 (see Table 7.1).

Table 7.1 Pain relief with bisphosphonates	
Time period	Proportion of patients with pain relief[+] [Odds ratio[*] (95% confidence interval dagger)]
Week 4	1.34: (0.96–1.85)
Week 8	2.52: (0.71–8.93)
Week 12	2.20: (1.36–3.50)
Best response within 12 weeks	1.87: (1.23–2.86)

[*] An odds ratio >1 favours the use of the intervention (bisphosphonate).

[+] A confidence interval (CI) that does not include 1 indicates that the effect is statistically significant, whereas a CI that includes 1 indicates that the effect is not significant.

The magnitude of pain relief was examined by looking at the mean pain scores over time. There was a trend for reduction in the mean pain score at 4 weeks (mean change −0.65/10: 95% CI: −2.77 to +1.46), and a statistically significant reduction in the mean pain score at 12 weeks (mean change −0.35/10: 95% CI: −0.39 to −0.31). Thus, the magnitude of benefit was modest to say the least.

Secondary endpoints, including the proportion of patients with analgesic reduction at 4, 8, and 12 weeks, and the mean analgesic scores support the conclusion of a moderate analgesic effect. Unfortunately, a quantitative summary of these effects was not possible, due to the variability in reporting outcomes. Sensitivity analyses examining methodological assumptions did not affect the conclusions of the analyses.

7.4.2 Results for different types of cancer

Of the 56 studies, 14 enrolled patients with bone metastases from any primary, 18 from breast cancer, 10 from multiple myeloma, 10 from prostate cancer, two with breast and multiple myeloma, and one with lung and other solid tumours. While a subgroup analysis was planned, too few trials containing the relevant information (proportion of patients with pain relief) were available to permit any conclusions to be drawn about whether a different effect is observed with different histologies.

7.4.3 Results for different bisphosphonates

Five randomized trials provided direct comparisons between different bisphosphonates. All of them compared pamidronate against a different bisphosphonate: three compared it with clodronate (Zhang et al., 1997; Diel et al., 1999; Jagdev et al., 2001), and two against zoledronate (Berenson et al., 2001; Rosen et al., 2001). A summary of the results of these studies is shown in Table 7.2.

Figure 7.2 Sensitivity analysis for site of primary: proportion of patients with pain relief (using best response within 12 weeks)

Comparison: 08 Sensitivity analysis
Outcome: 02 Primary disease site

Study	Treatment n/N	Control n/N	OR (95%Cl Random)
01 Breast			
Siris 1983	2/5	0/5	7.86[0.28,217.12]
Conte 1994	54/143	38/152	1.82[1.11,3.00]
Subtotal (95%Cl)	56/148	38/157	1.88[1.15,3.08]

Test for heterogeneity chi-square=0.73 df=1 p=0.39
Test for overall effect z=2.51 p=0.01

02 prostate			
Smith 1989	8/43	2/14	1.37[0.25,7.38]
Elomaa 1992	10/36	6/39	2.12[0.68,6.58]
Kylmala 1997	10/28	6/29	2.13[0.65,6.97]
Subtotal (95%Cl)	28/107	14/82	1.95[0.93,4.08]

Test for heterogeneity chi-square=0.21 df=2 p=0.9
Test for overall effect z=1.78 p=0.08

03 Multiple myeloma			
Heim 1995	25/77	19/80	1.54[0.77,3.11]
Mc Closkey 1998	53/264	54/272	1.01[0.66,1.55]
Subtotal(95%Cl)	78/341	73/352	1.14[0.79,1.64]

Test for heterogeneity chi-square=1.01 df=1 p=0.32
Test for overall effect z=0.68 p=0.5

04 Any primary			
Vinholes 1997a	5/25	1/27	6.50[0.70,60.14]
Arican 1999	26/33	5/17	8.91[2.34,33.91]
Subtotal(95%cl)	31/58	6/44	8.20[2.61,25.77]

Test for heterogeneity chi-square=0.06 df=1 p=0.81
Test for overall effect z=3.60 p=0.0003

| Total (95%Cl) | 193/654 | 131/635 | 1.87[1.23,2.86] |

Test for heterogeneity chi-square=13.95 df=8 p=0.083
Test for overall effect z=2.91 p=0.004

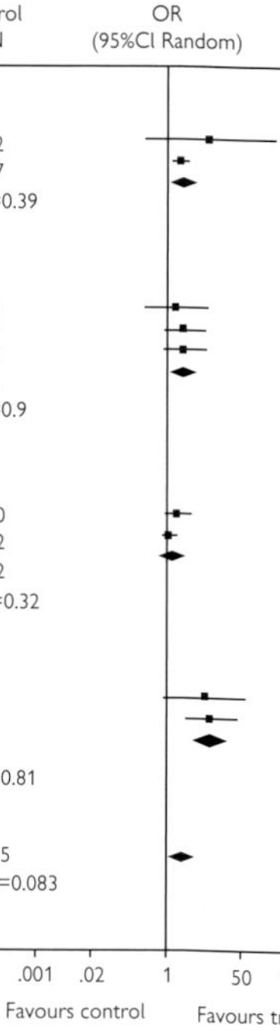

.001 .02 1 50 1000
Favours control   Favours treatment

Based on the limited data available, pamidronate appears to be a better choice than clodronate with a greater response rate, and a greater magnitude of pain relief. Further studies are necessary to elucidate the relative merits of pamidronate and the more potent bisphosphonates, such as ibandronate and zoledronate.

7.4.4 Bisphosphonates versus other treatment modalities

Comparisons between bisphosphonates and other treatment modalities are relatively uncommon. Indeed, only three randomized controlled trials have been published to date (Shucai et al., 1999; Wang et al., 2003; Wong et al., 2003). A summary of the results of these studies is shown in Table 7.3. It should be noted that the trials were generally underpowered.

Table 7.2	Randomized controlled trials comparing different bisphosphonates				
Study	Population	Bisphosphonate (1)	Bisphosphonate (2)	Outcomes	Comments
Zhang et al. (1997)	Any histology ECOG 0–2 Life expectancy >3 months n = 58	Pamidronate 30 mg i.v Single dose	Clodronate 300 mg i.v. 5 doses (5 days)	Proportion patients with pain relief at 7 days pamidronate group 63% (vs 39% clodronate group). Difference was significant (P < 0.05).	Difference in mean pain scores not significant
Diel et al. (1999)	Breast cancer n = 318	Pamidronate 60 mg i.v. (every 3 weeks)	Clodronate 2.4 g/day orally (continuously) or clodronate 900 mg i.v. (every 3 weeks)	Proportion patients with pain relief (time frame not specified) pamidronate group 30% (vs 15% oral clodronate group, and 25% i.v. clodronate group)	Study duration was 2 years
Jagdev et al. (2001)	Any histology n = 51	Pamidronate 90 mg i.v. (every 4 weeks)	Clodronate 1.6 g/day orally (continuously) or clodronate 1 g i.v. (loading dose) + clodronate 1.6 g/day orally (continuously)	Proportion of patients with pain relief at 3 months pamidronate group 56% (vs 18% oral clodronate group, and 25% i.v./oral clodronate group)	

Table 7.2 (Contd.)

Study	Population	Bisphosphonate (1)	Bisphosphonate (2)	Outcomes	Comments
Berenson et al. (2001)	Breast cancer Myeloma ECOG 0–2 Life expectancy >1 year n = 280	Pamidronate 90 mg i.v. (every 3–4 weeks)	Zoledronate 0.4 mg i.v. (every 4 weeks) or zoledronate 2 mg i.v. (every 4 weeks) or zoledronate 4 mg i.v. (every 4 weeks)	No pain data available within time frame of interest (12 weeks)	Study duration up to 1 year
Rosen et al. (2001)	Breast cancer Myeloma n = 1648	Pamidronate 90 mg i.v. (every 3–4 weeks)	Zoledronate 4 mg i.v. (every 3–4 weeks) or zoledronate 8 mg i.v. (every 3–4 weeks)	Reduction in median pain scores of 0.5 (0–10 NRS) at 12 weeks in both groups	Study duration was 1 year

7.5 **Clinical data tolerability**

Bisphosphonate side-effects commonly described include flu-like syndromes, and injection site reactions. Gastrointestinal toxicities, especially those associated with the oesophagus and stomach, have been of some concern (Lanza, 2002). However, randomized trials with standard doses did not identify excessive gastrointestinal toxicities.

Renal toxicity is another important area. Rapid infusions may result in renal toxicity, especially in patients with renal compromise. This necessitates restrictions on how quickly an intravenous infusion can be delivered (and on usage in patients with renal compromise). For example, pamidronate infusions (90 mg) are typically delivered over a period of 2 h, while zoledronate infusions (2 mg) are typically delivered over 15 min. However, ibandronate does not appear to possess the same renal toxicity concerns, and can be used in patients with varying degrees of renal impairment (Jackson, 2005; von Moos, 2005).

Adverse ocular events, including uveitis, scleritis and conjunctivitis have been reported with amino-bisphosphonate use, particularly pamidronate use (Leung *et al.*, 2005). A paper by Fraunfelder *et al.* (2003), based on reports submitted to the World Health Organization, US Food and Drug Administration and The National Registry of Drug Induced Ocular Side Effects, reported 17 cases of scleritis. Systemic steroids can be helpful, and, typically, the symptoms improve with discontinuation of the drug.

Bisphosphonate-associated osteonecrosis of the mandibular and maxillary bone has recently been described (Migliorati *et al.*, 2005). The pathophysiology of this condition is unknown, but the risk factors include dental extraction, local trauma, local infection and systemic chemotherapy. The condition has been reported with pamidronate and zoledronate, and usually appears after many months of treatment with these agents.

In the aforementioned systematic review, comparisons of bisphosphonate and placebo control arm toxicity profiles within eligible randomized trials were attempted. Identical categories were combined across trials. However, no attempt was made to pool together similar, but non-identical, categories across trials. A summary of the more common toxicity findings from randomized trials is described as follows.

Table 7.3 Randomized controlled trials comparing bisphosphonates with other treatment modalities

Study	Population	Bisphosphonate	Other modality	Outcomes	Comments
Shucai et al. (1999)	Single institution Lung cancer n = 80	Bonin + nothing or radiotherapy or chemotherapy	Radiotherapy alone (30–40 Gy, 3–5 Gy per fraction, 2–3 fractions per week, over 3–4 weeks)	Response rate bisphosphonate group: 88% (vs 83% other group). Difference not significant	Rationale for choosing additional modality in bisphosphonate group not specified
Wong et al. (2003)	Single institution Any histology n = 67	Pamidronate + radiotherapy (see next column)	Radiotherapy alone (8 Gy in 1 fraction, or 20 Gy in 5 fractions)	Response rate bisphosphonate group: 84% (vs 74% other group). Difference not significant	Time to response shorter in bisphosphonate group (difference not significant). Trial discontinued due to slow accrual
Wang et al. (2003)	Any histology n = 18	Pamidronate	Samarium-153	Proportion of patients with effective/excellent pain response within 3 weeks in bisphosphonate group: 44% (vs 78% other group)	

Clodronate

Forty toxicity categories have been cited in studies, including the following ones where there was a significantly higher risk in the bisphosphonate group:

(a) Diarrhoea or constipation: 5% patients in the active group versus 1% in the placebo group (OR: 3.34; 95% CI: 1.00–11.00).
(b) Hypocalcaemia: 5% patients in the active group versus 0% in the placebo group (OR: 6.0; 95% CI: 1.1–34.0).
(c) Elevated lactic dehydrogenase (LDH): elevated LDH was reported in one study, with 25/155 in the active group, and 0/156 in the control group, having an elevated LDH (Dearnaley et al., 2003). The clinical significance of an elevated LDH is unclear.

Pamidronate

Twenty-five different toxicity categories have been cited in studies, including:

(a) Fever: 13% patients in the active group versus 6% in the placebo group (OR: 2.3, 95% CI: 1.3–4.0).
(b) Hypocalcaemia: 4% patients in the active group versus 2% in the placebo group (OR: 2.5; 95% CI: 1.3–5.0).
(c) Discontinuation of therapy: 6% patients in the active group versus 2% in the placebo group (OR: 3.7; 95% CI: 1.0–13.5).

Zoledronate

Twenty-two toxicity categories have been cited in studies, including:

(a) Fever: 21% patients in the active group versus 13% in the placebo group (OR 1.77; 95% CI: 1.11–2.83).
(b) Deterioration in renal function: 18% patients in the active group versus 12% in the placebo group (OR: 1.70; 95% CI: 1.04–2.78). Elevated serum creatinine (grade 3) was seen in 4% patients receiving zoledronate, and 1% patients receiving placebo (OR: 4.70; 95% CI: 1.09–20.39).
(c) Nausea: 27% patients in the active group versus 18% in the placebo group (OR: 1.50; 95% CI: 1.20–1.90).
(d) Vomiting: 20% patients in the active group versus 13% in the placebo group (OR: 1.34; 95% CI: 1.00–1.77).

Ibandronate

Only one (Tripathy et al., 2004) of the two (Body et al., 2003; Tripathy et al., 2004) studies reported toxicity details. The toxicity profile was similar between the ibandronate and placebo groups, with slightly more treatment-related nausea, hypocalcaemia and abdominal pain in the ibandronate group. There was no increase in renal adverse effects.

7.6 **Conclusion**

Bisphosphonates delay the development of skeletal events, particularly in patients with breast cancer, multiple myeloma and prostate cancer. A positive effect of delaying these skeletal events is an overall reduction in pain secondary to bone resorption and its complications (e.g. pathological fracture, nerve compression). In addition, bisphosphonates also provide relief of bone pain, although the magnitude of the effect is modest in the short term (up to 12 weeks).

References

Berenson, J.R., Rosen, L.S., Howell, A. *et al.* (2001). Zoledronic acid reduces skeletal-related events in patients with osteolytic metastases. *Cancer*, **91**, 1191–200.

Bloomfield, D.J. (1998). Should bisphosphonates be part of the standard therapy of patients with multiple myeloma or bone metastases from other cancers? An evidence-based review. *J. Clin. Oncol.*, **16**, 1218–25.

Body, J.J., Diel, I.J., and Lichinitser, M.R. *et al.* (2003). Intravenous ibandronate reduces the incidence of skeletal complications in patients with breast cancer and bone metastases. *Ann. Oncol.*, **14**, 1399–405.

Dearnaley, D.P., Sydes, M.R., Mason, M.D. *et al.* (2003). A double-blind, placebo-controlled, randomized trial of oral sodium clodronate for metastatic prostate cancer (MRC PR05 Trial). *J. Natl Cancer Inst.*, **95**, 1300–11.

Dickersin, K., Scherer, R., and Lefebvre, C. (1994). Identifying relevant studies for systematic reviews. *BMJ*, **309**, 1286–91.

Diel, I.J., Marschner, N., Kindler, M. *et al.* (1999). Continual oral versus intravenous interval therapy with bisphosphonates in patients with breast cancer and bone metastases (Abstract 488). Proceedings of Annual Meeting of *Am. Soc. Clin. Oncol.*

Fleisch, H. (1987). Bisphosphonates—history and experimental basis. *Bone*, **8** (Suppl. 1), S23–8.

Fleisch, H., and Bisaz, S. (1962). Isolation from urine of pyrophosphate, a calcification inhibitor. *Am. J. Physiol.*, **203**, 671–5.

Fraunfelder, F.T., Fraunfelder, F.W., and Jensvold, B. (2003). Scleritis and other ocular side effects associated with pamidronate disodium. *Am. J. Opthalmol.*, **135**, 219–22.

Green, J.R. (2004). Bisphosphonates: preclinical review. *Oncologist*, **9**, (Suppl. 4), 3–13.

Jackson, G.H. (2005). Renal safety of ibandronate. *Oncologist*, **10** (Suppl. 1), 14–18.

Jadad, A.R., Moore, R.A., Carroll, D. *et al.* (1996). Assessing the quality of reports of randomized controlled trials: is blinding necessary? *Contr. Clin. Trials*, **17**, 1–12.

agdev, S.P., Purohit, P., Heatley, S., Herling, C., and Coleman, R.E. (2001). Comparison of the effects of intravenous pamidronate and oral clodronate on symptoms and bone resorption in patients with metastatic bone disease. *Ann. Oncol.*, **12**, 1433–8.

Krempien, R., Niethammer, A., Harms, W., and Debus, J. (2005). Bisphosphonates and bone metastases: current status and future directions. *Expert Rev.Anticancer Therapy*, **5**, 295–305.

Lanza, F.L. (2002). Gastrointestinal adverse effects of bisphosphonates: etiology, incidence and prevention. *Treatments Endocrinol.*, **1**, 37–43.

Leung, S., Ashar, B.H., and Miller, R.G. (2005). Bisphosphonate-associated scleritis: a case report and review. *Southern Med. J.*, **98**, 733–5.

Michaelson, M.D., and Smith, M.R. (2005). Bisphosphonates for treatment and prevention of bone metastases. *J. Clin. Oncol.*, **23**, 8219–24.

Migliorati, C.A., Schubert, M.M., Peterson, D.E., and Seneda, L.M. (2005). Bisphosphonate-associated osteonecrosis of mandibular and maxillary bone: an emerging oral complication of supportive cancer therapy. *Cancer*, **104**, 83–93.

Rosen, L.S., Gordon, D., Kaminski, M. *et al.* (2001). Zoledronic acid versus pamidronate in the treatment of skeletal metastases in patients with breast cancer or osteolytic lesions of multiple myeloma: a phase III, double-blind, comparative trial. *Cancer J.*, **7**, 377–87.

Rosen, L.S., Gordon, D., Tchekmedyian, S. *et al.* (2003). Zoledronic acid versus placebo in the treatment of skeletal metastases in patients with lung cancer and other solid tumors: a phase III, double-blind, randomized trial—the Zoledronic Acid Lung Cancer and Other Solid Tumors Study Group. *J. Clin. Oncol.*, **21**, 3150–7.

Santini, D., Vespasiani Gentilucci, U., Vincenzi, B. *et al.* (2003). The antineoplastic role of bisphosphonates: from basic research to clinical evidence. *Ann.Oncol.*, **14**, 1468–76.

Shucai, Z., Guimei, L., and Fanbin, H. (1999). (A clinical trial of Bonin in bone metastases of lung cancer). *Chinese J.Clin. Oncol.*, **26**, 445–7.

Small,E.J., Smith, M.R., Seaman, J.J., Petrone, S., and Kowalski, M.O. (2003). Combined analysis of two multicenter, randomized, placebo-controlled studies of pamidronate disodium for the palliation of bone pain in men with metastatic prostate cancer. *J. Clin. Oncol.*, **21**, 4277–84.

Stewart, A.F. (2005). Clinical practice. Hypercalcaemia associated with cancer. *New Engl. J. Med.*, **352**, 373–9.

Tripathy, D., Lichinitzer, M., Lazarev, A. *et al.* (2004). Oral ibandronate for the treatment of metastatic bone disease in breast cancer: efficacy and safety results from a randomized, double-blind, placebo-controlled trial. *Ann.Oncol.*, **15**, 743–50.

von Moos, R. (2005). Bisphosphonate treatment recommendations for oncologists. *Oncologist*, **10** (Suppl. 1), 19–24.

Wang, D.J., Liu, H.Q., Ren, J. *et al.* (2004). (Pamidronate in treatment of pain caused by bone metastasis). *Ai Zheng*, **23** (11 Suppl.), 1467–9.

Wang, R.F., Zhang, C.L., Zhu, S.L., and Zhu, M. (2003). A comparative study of samarium-153-ethylenediaminetetramethylene phosphonic acid with pamidronate disodium in the treatment of patients with painful metastatic bone cancer. *Med. Principles Pract.*, **12**, 97–101.

Wong, K., Franssen, E., Danjoux, C., and Bezjak, A. (2003). A randomized double blind placebo controlled trial of radiotherapy (XRT) with or without single dose Pamidronate (PAM) for pain relief in patients with painful bone metastases (Abstract 3099). Proceedings of Annual Meeting of *Am. Soc.Clin. Oncol.*

Wong, R., Shukla, V., Mensinkai, S., and Wiffen, P. (2004). Bisphosphonate agents for the management of pain secondary to bone metastases: a systematic review of effectiveness and safety. Technology Report Number 45. Canadian Coordinating Office for Health Technology Assessment, Ottawa.

Wong, R., and Wiffen, P.J. (2002). Bisphosphonates for the relief of pain secondary to bone metasatses. *Cochrane Database Syst. Rev.*, (2), CD002068.

Zhang, L., Guan, Z., and He, Y. (1997). (Randomized comparative clinical trial of treatment of bone metastatic diseases by infusion of pamidronate and clodronate). *Chinese J. Cancer*, **16**, 430–2.

Chapter 8

Radiotherapy

Nicholas van As and Robert Huddart

8.1 Introduction

Radiotherapy uses high energy X-rays, gamma rays, or electrons to deliver ionizing radiation to patients with malignant disease. There are three ways in which ionizing radiation can be delivered:

1. external beam therapy—using a machine such as a linear accelerator, or cobalt machine;

2. brachytherapy—using a localized radioisotope implant; or

3. radionuclide therapy—using a systemic radioisotope preparation.

External beam radiotherapy is by far the most commonly used modality in the management of bone pain: the most common type of treatment is local field radiotherapy, but wide field radiotherapy is also used in treating disseminated bone metastases. Radioisotopes are also used in treating disseminated bone metastases. However, there is no role for brachytherapy in the management of bone metastases.

This chapter will look at the evidence for the use of these different modalities of radiotherapy in the management of cancer-related bone pain.

8.2 Radiobiology

Radiation is the process in which a substance emits energy in the form of an electromagnetic wave. There is a vast spectrum of electromagnetic waves, with differing frequencies and wavelengths. The shorter the wavelength, the higher the chance of causing damage to tissues. At very short wavelengths, such as those used in radiotherapy, the phenomenon of ionization occurs: ionization is the actual ejection of an orbital electron from an atom, forming a pair of ions with opposite charges. Radiation passing through living cells will ionize the atoms and molecules within the cell.

Mechanism of cell damage

Ionizing radiation causes cellular damage by a number of different mechanisms (Steel, 2002). Radiation leads to the formation of free radicals and direct ionization of oxygen molecules. These, in turn, cause a variety of types of DNA damage. The most important lesions are irreparable double-strand breaks. DNA damage, which, when severe, leads to cell death, occurs in the both the tumour and the surrounding normal tissue.

An important concept when considering the effect of radiotherapy is the therapeutic index. The therapeutic index is the tumour response for a fixed level of normal tissue damage. The therapeutic window describes the possible difference between the tumour control dose and the normal tissue tolerance dose (Steel, 2002). Response rates to radiotherapy differ widely depending on tumour type (Emami et al., 1991).

Responses in normal tissue also vary from those that cause mild discomfort to others that are life-threatening. The speed at which the response occurs depends on both the tissue type being irradiated and the dose of radiation given in each fraction (Steel, 2002). Tissues that respond rapidly to radiotherapy are those which are rapidly dividing, including the haemopoietic cells and epithelial tissues. Those which respond late usually have a slow turnover, and include connective tissue and nerve cells (Steel, 2002). When assessing the risk of radiation damage to normal tissue, it is not only the total dose given, but also the fraction size that is important. Thus, as the fraction size increases, so the chance of late responding tissues being permanently damaged increases.

Mechanism of pain relief

Multiple clinical trials and systematic reviews have shown that radiotherapy is an effective modality for the palliation of painful bone metastases (Gaze et al., 1997; Hoskin, 1998; McQuay et al., 2000; Roos et al., 2000; Hoskin et al., 2001; Saarto et al., 2002; Roque et al., 2003). However, the mechanism of pain relief following radiotherapy is unclear: possible mechanisms include death of tumour cells, death of relevant host cells (e.g. macrophages), or activation and induction of cytokines involved in bone remodelling (e.g. transforming growth factor beta) (Anonymous, 1999).

Intuitively, it would seem likely that the tumour cell death would account for the pain relief that occurs following radiotherapy. However, several lines of evidence suggest that other mechanisms are involved: first, the primary tumour type does not seem to affect the rate of response (Price et al., 1986); second, research has shown little or no difference in response between 4 Gy single fraction and 8 Gy single fraction regimens, and between 8 Gy single fraction and 20 Gy multiple fraction regimens (Price et al., 1986; Hoskin et al., 1992; Anonymous, 1999).

Nevertheless, tumour shrinkage and bone healing are important when the aim of treatment is to reduce the risk of tumour progression leading to pathological fracture, or nerve root/spinal cord compression.

Healing with re-ossification occurs in the majority of lytic metastases following radiotherapy (65–80%) (Garmatis and Chu, 1978; Perez et al., 2003).

8.3 Local field radiotherapy

The aim of local field radiotherapy is to treat the area causing pain. As with all radiotherapy, the area is treated with a margin of normal tissue to allow for inaccuracies in set-up, and for patient movement. In palliative radiotherapy for bone metastases, the margins are usually generous as the patients are generally less fit and in pain, which makes them more likely to move between set-up and treatment (and the dose to normal tissues is not likely to cause problems).

Dose/fractionation

In 1999 the Cochrane group reviewed the use of radiotherapy for painful bone metastases. The review included data from 20 randomized controlled trials; 15 other studies were excluded for various methodological reasons. The trials were not sufficiently alike to allow pooling of data and therefore no meta-analysis was performed. Nevertheless, the authors concluded that radiotherapy provides effective analgesia for painful metastases. Thus, over 40% of patients could expect ≥ 50% pain relief at 1 month, and 30% could expect complete relief (McQuay et al., 2000). There was no discernible difference between fractionation schedules, or between different doses using the same schedule. (The authors did not recommend a standard fractionation regimen.)

In 1999 a further study was conducted on behalf of the Bone Pain Trial Working Group (Anonymous, 1999). The study compared treatment with an 8 Gy single fraction and a multiple fraction regimen of either 20 Gy in five fractions, or 30 Gy in 10 fractions (98% of patients in the multiple fraction arm received 20 Gy in five fractions, and only 2% patients received 30 Gy in 10 fractions). Patients recorded pain severity and analgesic requirements on a self-assessment questionnaire before treatment, at 2 weeks, monthly for 6 months, and then 2-monthly until 1 year after radiotherapy. The primary endpoint was pain relief. In total, 765 patients were entered into the study. Overall, 78% of patients in both the single fraction arm and the multiple fraction arm experienced pain relief at some point following radiotherapy. Complete response was defined as being pain-free with no increase in analgesic requirement: complete response was reported in 57% of patients in the single fraction arm, and 58% patients in the multiple fraction arm. There was no difference between the arms in the time to first improvement in pain, time to complete pain relief, or time to increase in pain at any time over the 12 month period. There was also no difference in the acute toxicity of a single fraction of 8 Gy and the multiple fraction regimens. Although re-treatment was more common in the single fraction arm, this was felt possibly to be due to clinicians being more likely to re-treat after a single fraction than after a multiple fraction regimen (Anonymous, 1999).

The aforementioned study (Anonymous, 1999) and earlier studies (Nielson et al., 1998; Price et al., 1986) have shown that a single fraction of 8 Gy is an effective and safe treatment for bone pain due to metastases. However, despite these studies, there is still no international consensus on how many fractions to use. In the USA most clinicians use 10 fractions, in Canada the most common regimen used is 20 Gy in five fractions, whereas in the UK most clinicians use an 8 Gy single fraction (Chow et al., 2000; Lievens et al., 2000). In our view the equal efficacy, patient convenience, and lower cost should make a single 8 Gy fraction the standard treatment for palliation of pain from bone metastases.

Side effects

Usually the side-effects of radiotherapy for bone pain are mild. A proportion of patients will report that the pain gets worse for a short period before it improves ('pain flare'). Chow et al. (2005) studied 88 patients being treated with radiotherapy for bone pain, and found that 14% had a pain flare on the day following the radiotherapy. Pain flares are normally easily controlled with additional analgesics and/or corticosteroids.

Other side-effects are specific to the area irradiated. The unwanted effects of palliative radiotherapy are often due to the exit dose of radiotherapy. An example of this occurs when irradiating the lower thoracic spine; a proportion of the radiation will pass through the stomach, which may lead to the development of nausea and vomiting. It is important to think about the exit path of the radiation beam, so that appropriate prophylactic medications can be given.

The side-effects are usually limited to the treated area. However, fatigue is a common systemic symptom occurring in 60–90% of patients who receive a course of radiotherapy (Visovsky and Schneider, 2003). The incidence of fatigue following radiotherapy for bone pain is not known. The pathophysiology of fatigue following radiotherapy is poorly understood, but is probably multifactorial in origin (Visovsky and Schneider, 2003; Lawrence et al., 2004).

Re-treatment

Mithal et al. (1994) conducted a retrospective analysis of patients who were retreated with palliative radiotherapy for bone metastases. The overall response rate to the initial treatment was 84%, and to the first re-treatment was 87%. In addition, seven out of eight patients achieved good pain relief after being treated for a third time.

The decision regarding re-treating previously irradiated sites is essentially one of balancing the benefits of treating the tumour over the risks of re-treating the normal tissues. In most cases, there are no concerns about re-treating the bone disease. However, there are concerns about re-treating the spine, because of the spinal cord's tolerance for radiotherapy. Nevertheless, recent data suggest that it may be relatively safe to retreat the spine/spinal cord (Rades et al., 2005).

8.4 **Wide field radiotherapy**

Wide field radiotherapy can be done in several ways including radiation to the entire upper half of the body, radiation to the entire lower half of the body, radiation to the mid-section (from the lower chest to the upper thighs), and sequential hemi-body radiation in which half of the body is irradiated in one session and the other half of the body is irradiated in a later session (4–6 weeks later). The latter procedure allows enough time for the bone marrow from the un-irradiated half of the body to re-populate the marrow cavity in the irradiated half of the body.

Wide field radiotherapy can be used as a single modality for widespread painful bone metastases, or as an adjunct to local field radiotherapy in order to reduce the risk of pain developing in other known or occult bone metastases.

Dose/fractionation

Wide field radiotherapy can either be given in a single fraction, or a fractionated regimen. The optimal dose for a single fraction is 8 Gy to the lower half of the body, and 6 Gy to the upper half of the body (Salazar et al., 1986). The reason for the lower dose to the upper half of the body is the risk of lung toxicity with this type of treatment.

Reported response rates for wide-field radiotherapy vary from 64 to 100% (Nag and Shah, 1986; Salazar et al., 1986; Kuban et al., 1989; Quilty et al., 1994). However, these studies tended to involve relatively small numbers of patients, and the methods of assessing pain were not always clearly stated. Salazar et al. showed that fractionated wide field radiotherapy (15 Gy in five fractions over 1 week) was more effective than single fraction regimens, but with a similar overall toxicity profile (Salazar et al., 1986, 1996).

A trial conducted on behalf of the Radiation Therapy Oncology Group compared local field radiotherapy alone to local field radiotherapy with the addition of hemi-body radiotherapy. This trial essentially demonstrated a delayed time to disease progression, an increased time to development of new disease, and when prostate patients were analysed separately, a trend towards survival benefit at 1 year, in the experimental group (Poulter et al., 1992). One major problem with this study was a high rate of protocol violations in the experimental group. Thus, only 70% of the patients assigned to receive hemi-body radiotherapy actually received the treatment. Furthermore, the results were not analysed on an intention-to-treat basis. There were significantly higher rates of (transient) haematological toxicity in the group who received hemi-body radiotherapy.

Side effects

Wide field radiotherapy can cause significant nausea, and patients need to be well hydrated and given appropriate anti-emetic cover prior to treatment. This should include a $5HT_3$ receptor antagonist. Wide field radiotherapy can also cause bone marrow suppression, and so patients with markedly impaired bone marrow function should not receive this type of treatment.

Wide field radiotherapy is not commonly used in the UK. There are probably a number of reasons for this phenomenon, including increasing use of alternative treatment strategies, increasing use of myelosuppressive chemotherapy (see above), and misperceptions about the relative toxicity of this form of treatment.

8.5 **Radioisotopes**

A number of radioisotopes have been used in the treatment of bone metastases (e.g. phosphorus-32, strontium-89, samarium-153, rhenium-186). Most of these radioisotopes are beta emitters: a beta particle is an unpaired, singly charged, electron possessing kinetic energy. Beta particles travel for a short distance within tissue leading to damage of cells within close proximity.

Phosphorus-32 (^{32}P)

The first isotope to be used was radioactive phosphorus. It was widely used until the 1980s when newer agents were developed: it is as effective in providing pain relief as newer agents, but is associated with more haematological toxicity than the newer agents (pancytopenia) (Silberstein, 1993; Pandit-Taskar et al., 2004).

Strontium-89 (^{89}Sr)

Strontium-89 is an analogue of calcium, and it concentrates in osteoblastic bone metastases. After intravenous injection, 50% of the activity is deposited in the bone, where it may remain for up to 100 days (Perez et al., 2004). The unabsorbed agent is excreted in urine. There are a number of trials that have looked at the use of strontium for treating bone pain. However, most of these trials have only included patients with metastatic prostate cancer.

Lewington et al. (1991) conducted a randomized, double-blind, cross-over trial comparing a single intravenous dose of ^{89}Sr with placebo in patients with metastatic prostate cancer. The response was assessed at 5 weeks after treatment: the assessment involved patients' self-assessment of pain, analgesic consumption, incidence of new pain points, and incidence of side-effects. The results showed a statistically significant benefit for ^{89}Sr over placebo therapy.

Porter et al. (1993) conducted a randomized, double-blind study comparing the addition of a single dose of either ^{89}Sr or placebo after local field radiotherapy in patients with prostate cancer. There was no difference noted in relief of pain at the index site of treatment. However, there was a statistically significant improvement in quality of life, and a reduction in the intake of analgesics, in the arm treated with ^{89}Sr. Furthermore, there was a statistically significant reduction in progression of disease, as measured by sites of new pain, or the requirement for further radiotherapy, in the arm treated with ^{89}Sr. Not surprisingly, marrow toxicity was greater in the ^{89}Sr arm.

Quilty et al. (1994) compared the use of local field radiotherapy or hemi-body radiotherapy and ^{89}Sr. All treatments provided effective pain relief, and there was no statistically significant difference between the treatment modalities. Thus, at 3 months, 61% patients treated with local field radiotherapy, 64% of patients treated with hemi-body radiotherapy, and 66% treated with ^{89}Sr, reported sustained improvement in pain. However, more patients reported new pain sites after local field radiotherapy or hemi-body radiotherapy than after ^{89}Sr therapy.

Samarium-153 (^{153}Sm)

^{153}Sm has an affinity for bone, and it concentrates in areas of bone turnover: it binds to hydroxyapatite, and it binds predominantly in osteoblastic lesions (Perez et al., 2004). The ratio of binding in osteoblastic tissue is 6:1 as compared to normal bone (Perez et al., 2004). There are a couple of randomized controlled trials involving ^{153}Sm. In these trials the majority of patients had either prostate or breast cancer, had failed all systemic options, and had undergone maximal external beam radiotherapy.

Resche et al. (1997) demonstrated that ^{153}Sm provided at least some relief in 70% of patients at 4 weeks after treatment. Treatment with ^{153}Sm produced improvement from baseline in all patient-rated efficacy assessments, including degree of pain, pain relief, and quality of sleep. Female patients with breast cancer had the most noticeable improvement. The toxicity of the treatment was predictable bone marrow suppression with no episodes of febrile neutropenia or toxic deaths.

Serafini et al. (1998) randomized patients to receive either 0.50 mCi/kg of ^{153}Sm, 1 mCi/kg of ^{153}Sm, or placebo. In those patients that received the 1.0 mCi/kg dose, pain relief was observed in 62–72% during the first 4 weeks, with marked or complete relief noted in 31% by week 4. Furthermore, in those patients who received the 1.0 mCi/kg dose, persistence of pain relief was seen in 43% through to week 16. Bone marrow suppression was mild, and reversible, in this study.

Radionuclides are not widely used in the UK, despite the afore-mentioned studies showing that they are effective in improving bone pain (particularly in patients with prostate cancer). There are a number of possible reasons for this phenomenon:

- frailty of patients
- contra-indications to treatment (see below)
- availability of other treatments for cancer, e.g. chemotherapy
- availability of other treatments for pain, e.g. bisphosphonates
- expense of treatment: ^{89}Sr costs ~£1300 per treatment.

There are a number of well-recognized contra-indications to treatment with radioisotopes (Perez et al., 2004). These include pathological fracture or impending fracture, spinal cord compression or impending cord compression, hypercalcaemia, anaemia (i.e. persistent anaemia), thrombocytopaenia (i.e. platelet count <100). The reason that isotopes are contraindicated in actual or impending fractures is that the isotope remains present in the bone for months after administration, and so would be a radioactive hazard if surgery were required during this period.

References

Anonymous (1999). 8 Gy single fraction radiotherapy for the treatment of metastatic skeletal pain: randomised comparison with a multifraction schedule over 12 months of patient follow-up. Bone Pain Trial Working Party. *Radiother. Oncol.*, **52**, 111–21.

Chow, E., Danjoux, C., Wong, R. et al. (2000). Palliation of bone metastases: a survey of patterns of practice among Canadian radiation oncologists. *Radiother.Oncol.*, **56**, 305–14.

Chow, E., Ling, A., Davis, L., Panzarella, T., and Danjoux, C. (2005). Pain flare following external beam radiotherapy and meaningful change in pain scores in the treatment of bone metastases. *Radiother. Oncol.*, **75**, 64–9.

Emami, B., Lyman, J., Brown, A. et al. (1991). Tolerance of normal tissue to therapeutic irradiation. *Int. J. Radiat. Oncol., Biol., Phys.*, **21**, 109–22.

Garmatis, C.J., and Chu, F.C. (1978). The effectiveness of radiation therapy in the treatment of bone metastases from breast cancer. *Radiology*, **126**, 235–7.

Gaze, M.N., Kelly, C.G., Kerr, G.R. et al. (1997). Pain relief and quality of life following radiotherapy for bone metastases: a randomised trial of two fractionation schedules. *Radiother. Oncol.*, **45**, 109–16.

Hoskin, P.J. (1988). Scientific and clinical aspects of radiotherapy in the relief of bone pain. *Cancer Surv.*, **7**, 69–86.

Hoskin, P.J., Price, P., Easton, D. et al. (1992). A prospective randomised trial of 4 Gy or 8 Gy single doses in the treatment of metastatic bone pain. *Radiother. Oncol.*, **23**, 74–8.

Hoskin, P.J., Yarnold, J.R., Roos, D.R., and Bentzen, S. (2001). Radiotherapy for bone metastases. *Clin. Oncol. (R. Coll. Radiol.)*, **13**, 88–90.

Kuban, D.A., Delbridge, T., el-Mahdi, A.M., and Schellhammer, P.F. (1989). Half-body irradiation for treatment of widely metastatic adenocarcinoma of the prostate. *J. Urol.*, **141**, 572–4.

Lawrence, D.P., Kupelnick, B., Miller, K., Devine, D., and Lau, J. (2004). Evidence report on the occurrence, assessment, and treatment of fatigue in cancer patients. *J. Nat. Cancer Inst.. Monogr.*, (32), 40–50.

Lewington, V.J., McEwan, A.J., Ackery, D.M. et al. (1991). A prospective, randomised double-blind crossover study to examine the efficacy of strontium-89 in pain palliation in patients with advanced prostate cancer metastatic to bone. *Eur. J. Cancer*, **27**, 954–8.

Lievens, Y., Kesteloot, K., Rijnders, A., Kutcher, G., and Van den Bogaert, W. (2000). Differences in palliative radiotherapy for bone metastases within Western European countries. *Radiother. Oncol.*, **56**, 297–303.

McQuay, H.J., Collins, S.L., Carroll, D., and Moore, R.A. (2000). Radiotherapy for the palliation of painful bone metastases. *Cochrane Database Syst. Rev.*, (2), CD001793.

Mithal, N.P., Needham, P.R., and Hoskin, P.J. (1994). Retreatment with radiotherapy for painful bone metastases. *Int. J. Radiat. Oncol., Biol., Phys.*, **29**, 1011–4.

Nag, S., and Shah, V. (1986). Once-a-week lower hemibody irradiation (HBI) for metastatic cancers. *Int. J. Radiat. Oncol., Biol., Phys.*, **12**, 1003–5.

Nielsen, O.S., Bentzen, S.M., Sandberg, E., Gadeberg, C.C., and Timothy, A.R. (1998). Randomized trial of single dose versus fractionated palliative radiotherapy of bone metastases. *Radiother. Oncol.*, **47**, 233–40.

Pandit-Taskar, N., Batraki, M., and Divgi, C.R. (2004). Radiopharmaceutical therapy for palliation of bone pain from osseous metastases. *J. Nucl. Med.*, **45**, 1358–65.

Perez, C., Brady, L.W., Halperin, C., and Schmidt-Ulrich R (2003). *Principles and practice of radiation oncology*. Lippincott/Williams & Wilkins, Philadelphia.

Porter, A.T., McEwan, A.J., Powe, J.E. et al. (1993). Results of a randomized phase-III trial to evaluate the efficacy of strontium-89 adjuvant to local field external beam irradiation in the management of endocrine resistant metastatic prostate cancer. *Int. J. Radiat. Oncol., Biol., Phys.*, **25**, 805–13.

Poulter, C.A., Cosmatos, D., and Rubin, P. et al. (1992). A report of RTOG 8206: a phase III study of whether the addition of single dose hemibody irradiation to standard fractionated local field irradiation is more effective than local field irradiation alone in the treatment of symptomatic osseous metastases. *Int. J. Radiat. Oncol., Biol., Phys.*, **23**, 207–14.

83

Price, P., Hoskin, P.J., Easton, D., Austin, D., Palmer, S.G., and Yarnold, J.R. (1986). Prospective randomised trial of single and multifraction radiotherapy schedules in the treatment of painful bony metastases. *Radiother. Oncol.*, **6**, 247–55.

Quilty, P.M., Kirk, D., Bolger, J.J. et al. (1994) A comparison of the palliative effects of strontium-89 and external beam radiotherapy in metastatic prostate cancer. *Radiother. Oncol.*, **31**, 33–40.

Rades, D., Stalpers, L.J., Veninga, T., and Hoskin, P.J. (2005). Spinal reirradiation after short-course RT for metastatic spinal cord compression. *Int. J. Radiat. Oncol., Biol., Phys.*, **63**, 872–5.

Resche, I., Chatal, J.F., Pecking, A. et al. (1997). A dose-controlled study of 153Sm-ethylenediaminetetramethylenephosphonate (EDTMP) in the treatment of patients with painful bone metastases. *Eur. J. Cancer*, **33**, 1583–91.

Roos, D.E., O'Brien, P.C., Smith, J.G. et al. (2000). A role for radiotherapy in neuropathic bone pain: preliminary response rates from a prospective trial (Trans-tasman radiation oncology group, TROG 96.05). *Int. J. Radiat. Oncol., Biol., Phys.*, **46**, 975–81.

Roque, M., Martinez, M.J., Alonso, P., Catala, E., Garcia, J.L., and Ferrandiz, M. (2003). Radioisotopes for metastatic bone pain. *Cochrane Database Syst. Rev.*, (4), CD003347.

Saarto, T., Janes, R., Tenhunen, M., and Kouri, M. (2002). Palliative radiotherapy in the treatment of skeletal metastases. *Eur. J. Pain*, **6**, 323–30.

Salazar, O.M., Rubin, P., Hendrickson, F.R. et al. (1986). Single-dose half-body irradiation for palliation of multiple bone metastases from solid tumors. Final Radiation Therapy Oncology Group report. *Cancer*, **58**, 29–36.

Salazar, O.M., Damotta, N.W., Bridgman, S.M., Cardiges, N.M. and Slawson, R.G. (1996) Fractionated half-body irradiation for pain palliation in widely metastatic cancers: comparison with single dose. *Int. J. Radiat. Oncol., Biol., Phys.*, **36**, 49–60.

Serafini, A.N., Houston, S.J., Resche, I. et al. (1998). Palliation of pain associated with metastatic bone cancer using samarium-153 lexidronam: a double-blind placebo-controlled clinical trial. *J. Clin. Oncol.*, **16**, 1574–81.

Silberstein, E.B. (1993). The treatment of painful osseous metastases with phosphorus-32-labeled phosphates. *Semin. Oncol.*, **20** (Suppl. 2), 10–21.

Steel, G.G. (2002). *Basic clinical radiobiology* (3rd edn). Hodder Arnold, London.

Visovsky, C., and Schneider, S.M. (2003). Cancer-related fatigue. *Online J. Iss. Nurs.*, **8**, 8.

Chapter 9

Anaesthetic and interventional techniques

Paul Farquhar-Smith

9.1 Introduction

The World Health Organization (WHO, 1996) guidelines for the treatment of cancer pain are a widely accepted therapeutic tool. It has been suggested that the WHO ladder (see Figure 4.2), used as part of a multidisciplinary approach to analgesia, controls pain in >80% cancer patients, and in 75% of those in the terminal stages of disease (Bruera and Kim, 2003).

Interventional approaches are viewed by some correspondents as a further step on the WHO ladder (Figure 9.1) (Miguel, 2000). However, interventional techniques should not be seen as a separate entity, but as part of an integrated approach to pain control in bone pain. Thus, even before the WHO ladder approach has failed, interventional input may be warranted to control pain.

This chapter will focus upon specific/relevant interventional techniques such as neuraxial delivery of opioids and local anaesthetics, local anaesthetic and neurolytic peripheral nerve blocks, and direct bone tumour ablation. It should be noted that much of the available data on these techniques refers to patients with non-cancer pain (rather than cancer pain). Readers are advised to consult one of the many comprehensive textbooks on pain or palliative medicine for further details about these and other interventional techniques (Breivik et al., 2002; Doyle et al., 2004; McMahon and Koltzenburg, 2005).

9.2 Neuraxial drug delivery

Neuraxial drug delivery includes intrathecal (also referred to as spinal or subarachnoid) and epidural approaches. Intrathecal administration delivers drugs into the cerebrospinal fluid within the subarachnoid space, where they can act directly on the spinal cord. In contrast, epidural administration requires the opioid or local

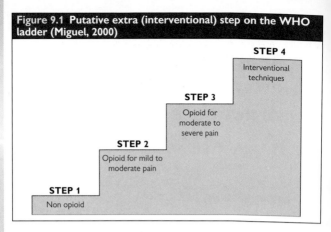

Figure 9.1 Putative extra (interventional) step on the WHO ladder (Miguel, 2000)

STEP 4
Interventional techniques

STEP 3
Opioid for moderate to severe pain

STEP 2
Opioid for mild to moderate pain

STEP 1
Non opioid

anaesthetic to diffuse across the dura mater in order to reach the spinal cord. Both routes reduce systemic exposure and therefore potentially minimize central side-effects.

The three most common sites of metastatic bony spread are the vertebrae, pelvis and femora (Kori et al., 1997), all of which are susceptible to neuraxial blockade (even if multiple sites are affected). Indeed, neuraxial blockade may be the only respite from incident pain secondary to pathological fractures, and can provide necessary analgesia before relevant orthopaedic intervention.

Neuraxial opioids, with or without local anaesthetic, are efficacious in cancer pain management, and may have advantages over oral administration. For example, Vainio and Tigerstedt (1988) reported that epidural opioids for cervical or lumbar plexus pain were associated with fewer side-effects than oral opioids, and that there was no difference in pain scores between the routes. Similarly, Kalso et al. (1996) reported that patients required less self-titrated epidural morphine than subcutaneous morphine, and that both routes produced the same analgesic efficacy. In this study, both routes provided better pain control, and fewer side-effects, than historical oral morphine controls.

Rauck et al. (2003) demonstrated improved pain scores after intrathecal opioid delivery in cancer pain patients with refractory pain, or uncontrollable side-effects, although the lack of a control group weakens the veracity of the conclusions of the study. A more recent investigation examined patients with refractory pain (defined as pain scores of ≥5/10 and receiving ≥200 mg / day morphine or equivalent), randomized to either 'comprehensive medical management' (all pain management strategies, except intrathecal opioids and neurosurgical intervention), and comprehensive medical management plus an implantable spinal drug delivery system (Smith et al., 2005). The use of intrathecal opioids was associated with lower pain scores, fewer side effects, and an increased survival. However, some authors have raised methodological concerns about this study (Davis et al., 2005).

The benefits of neuraxial delivery are at a 'cost' of increased levels of intervention and potential side-effects. Spinal and epidural infusions necessitate close liaison between anaesthetic and other services, and require increased intensity of medical and nursing input. Complications related to catheter insertion include epidural haematoma, epidural abscess formation and meningitis. Although rare, these adverse events can cause irreversible neurological deficit, and the infective complications may also be life-threatening.

Opioids

Historically, morphine and diamorphine have been used most frequently both epidurally and intrathecally. Nevertheless, the shorter-acting fentanyl is now also widely used. Recently epidural oxycodone had been shown to be as efficacious as epidural morphine, with lower rates of nausea, vomiting and pruritus, in patients with non-malignant pain (Yanagidate and Dohi, 2004).

The effective epidural and intrathecal dose of opioid is less when compared to systemic opioids, due to delivery of opioid in close proximity to spinal opioid receptors. However, neuraxial opioids can still cause side-effects such as sedation, nausea and vomiting, decreased gut motility and pruritus. Moreover, neuraxial delivery of hydrophilic opioids such as morphine risks cranial spread, and (late onset) respiratory depression.

Local anaesthetics and other agents

Local anaesthetics, such as bupivacaine and lidocaine, are used synergistically with opioids to reduce opioid requirements. Local anaesthetics may also be required for pains that are poorly responsive to opioids. Local anaesthetics depend on concentration and volume for their effect: increasing the volume increases the dermatome spread, whilst increasing the concentration increases the density of block and makes muscle weakness more likely.

Although the ideal is to reduce pain without numbness or weakness, some bony pains require high concentrations of local anaesthetics that make these side-effects more likely. Higher concentrations also risk sphincter disturbance, resulting in urinary retention and possibly faecal incontinence. Neuraxial delivery is appropriate for pain below the T4 dermatome: higher blocks can cause upper limb weakness, excessive sympathetic block to the heart (and hypotension), and possibly diaphragmatic paralysis.

Neuraxial administration of other analgesic agents has also been employed in the treatment of cancer-related bone pain. For example, epidural clonidine (an α_2 agonist) has been shown to be effective in reducing cancer pain inadequately controlled with opioids (Eisenach et al., 1995).

Route of administration

Historically, the epidural route has been more widely used than the intrathecal route. Nevertheless, intrathecal infusions are becoming more widespread, and are the neuraxial technique of choice in several centres (Nitescu et al., 2003).

A literature review compared the efficacies, complications and failure rates of epidural or intrathecal treatment in refractory non-malignant pain (Dahm et al., 1998): intrathecal administration was associated with better pain relief, and lower rates of complications, than epidural administration. However, there was no methodological assessment or grading of the quality of the studies incorporated in the review. Nitescu et al., (1990) reported on 25 patients with advanced cancer, who were switched to intrathecal infusion after failure of epidural infusion of morphine and bupivacaine: pain control improved, and lower doses of morphine and bupivicaine were required, following the switch.

Intrathecal infusion may be preferable in patients with concomitant epidural metastatic disease. Intuitively, epidural tumour would be expected to interfere with both catheter positioning, and with the spread of injectate, and so potentially to affect the quality of block. Infusion of high opioid concentrations into the subarachnoid space has also been associated with catheter tip inflammatory masses that may result in neurological sequelae (Peng and Massicotte, 2004).

A retrospective study of 201 consecutive intrathecal infusions observed that patients with epidural metastases and spinal stenosis required higher doses of opioid and bupivicaine than those without epidural disease (Appelgren et al., 1997). Moreover, four unexpected paraplegias occurred in this series of intrathecal infusions. Thus, although epidural disease is an indication for an intrathecal approach, it is still associated with higher risks.

The choice of neuraxial technique will depend upon careful consideration of diverse patient and practitioner factors, such as the presence of epidural disease and local experience and training of the medical and nursing staff.

Type of system

Both external and implantable systems can be used for epidural and intrathecal administration of opioids and local anaesthetics. Implantable systems require operative insertion, and are more expensive when compared to external pumps (Lawson and Siemaszko, 2003). Some authors state that implantable systems become cost-effective after 3 months (Bedder et al., 1991), whilst others claim the 'cross-over' occurs after 6–7 months (Erdine and Talu, 1998). The decision to use an implantable system is therefore influenced by the prognosis of the patient.

9.1.1 Epidural steroid injection

Although most of the data concerning the efficacy of epidural steroid injections relates to non-malignant pain, there are certain commonalities that support extrapolation of the evidence to a bone cancer population.

A recent review by the American Society of Interventional Pain Physicians has weighed the existing evidence for interventional techniques in chronic spinal pain (Boswell et al., 2005). Evidence for the efficacy of epidural steroid injections for lumbar radiculopathy (pain secondary to nerve root irritation) was described as 'strong' for short-term relief, and 'limited' for long-term relief. Similarly, the efficacy of caudal epidural steroid injections for lower back pain and radiculopathy was supported by 'strong' evidence in the short term, and 'moderate' evidence in the long term.

Bone cancer patients can have radiculopathy secondary to direct tumour involvement, or vertebral invasion and vertebral collapse. Thus, in patients with signs of radiculopathy, a lumbar or caudal epidural steroid injection may be of benefit. (MRI is often used to assess nerve root impingement and epidural disease.)

There are limited data on the efficacy of epidural steroid injections for bone pain per se (i.e. without evidence of radiculopathy). However, lack of evidence of efficacy is not the same as evidence of lack of efficacy, and the popularity of epidural steroid injection suggests a significant benefit. It is unclear, however, what advantage epidural steroids may have over high-dose systemic steroids.

9.2 Peripheral nerve blocks

9.2.1 Local anaesthetic nerve blocks

In theory, bone pain in the distribution of any peripheral nerve can be blocked. In cancer pain patients, the most common blocks are intercostal nerve blocks (for pain from rib metastases), paravertebral blocks (for pain from more extensive rib metastases), and brachial plexus blocks (for pain from upper limb metastases) (Reale et al., 2001). Lower limb nerves can be blocked, although neuraxial techniques may be preferred in this situation.

There is little evidence other than anecdotal and case report studies to support the efficacy of these interventions in both cancer and non-cancer pain (de Leon-Casasola, 2004). Nevertheless nerve blocks are widely used, and with careful patient selection can be efficacious (Reale et al., 2001; Kim, 2005). Current practice involves the routine use of a peripheral nerve stimulator to confirm correct needle placement.

Local anaesthetics block nerve conduction in a reversible manner. The duration of conduction block is directly related to the duration of the local anaesthetics. However, there is some evidence to suggest that blocking the pain transmission can 'break the cycle' and result in analgesia that outlasts the expected duration of local anaesthetic action (Arner et al., 1990). This tenet is supported by current knowledge about plasticity of pain processing: interruption of pain afferent input to the spinal cord by local anaesthetic block could reduce mechanisms of central sensitization that are thought to be important in chronic pain states (Coderre et al., 1993). There may be increased effect with repeated blocks (Arner et al., 1990).

Steroids have been used in an attempt to prolong the action of local anaesthetic nerve blocks, putatively by reducing perineural inflammation. The implication is that if there is not an inflammatory component to the pain, then the steroid will not be efficacious in this situation.

Continuous infusion of local anaesthetic via a peripheral nerve catheter can prolong the analgesic action (Fischer et al., 1996). However, the evidence for the efficacy of continuous infusions in bone pain is again anecdotal or from case reports (Khor and Ditton, 1996). Indwelling perineural catheters are associated with increased risk of infection, and the possibility of local anaesthetic overdose.

Infrequently, opioids are added to local anaesthetic infusions to improve the analgesic effect (Nishikawa et al., 2000), by virtue of an action on peripheral opioid receptors (Janson and Stein, 2003).

9.2.2 Neurolytic nerve blocks

Neurolytic nerve blocks can be employed to give longer-lasting benefit (Lamacraft and Cousins, 1997). They are predominantly used for cancer pain patients, where pain relief benefits may outweigh the disadvantages of nerve damage. Patient selection is critical, and yet there is little evidence to guide this decision.

An effective neurolytic block will cause numbness in the nerve's receptive field, and may be associated with late onset 'reafferentation' (neuropathic) pain. Alcohol (50–100%), or phenol (e.g. 7%), are used to cause neurolysis. Alcohol causes more pain on injection, and may be associated with more late-onset pain (Lordon, 2002). Phenol requires the use of glass syringes, and is potentially more damaging to neighbouring structures (although may spare adjacent motor nerve fibres). Phenol may not be as damaging for the nerve cell body, and hence is associated with more rapid axonal regrowth, resulting in both earlier recurrence of the original pain and the earlier development of reafferentation pain. Phenol also has potentially harmful systemic side-effects.

Intercostal nerve neurolysis is the most common block used for bone pain, but successful paravertebral neurolysis has also been documented (Antila and Kirvela, 1998). Neurolysis should only follow a successful local anaesthetic block. However, although the lack of analgesia from local anaesthetic injection generally predicts the failure of a neurolytic block, a good result after local anaesthetic injection does not guarantee the success of subsequent chemical destruction.

Neurolysis can also be achieved either by freezing with cryoanalgesia, or by heating using radiofrequency lesioning (Miguel, 2000). Cryolesioning is generally safe, although it is shorter-lasting than the other neurolytic procedures; it has little capacity for post-procedural reafferentation pain, due to preservation of the nerve's neurolemma (Miguel, 2000). Both of these interventions require specialist expertise and equipment.

Spinal neurolysis has also been used for severe terminal cancer pain, again supported by anecdotes and case reports, rather than by controlled trials (Candido and Stevens, 2003). Chemical posterior rhizotomy by intrathecal phenol has been used to ablate the dorsal horn of the spinal cord, and so disrupt nociceptive impulses (Swerdlow, 1978). The risk of collateral damage to motor and sphincter function limits this technique to patients with intractable pain and a poor prognosis. Less extensive, but still able to cause similar complications, is the neurolytic saddle block, which is occasionally used for intractable pelvic pain, including pain of bony origin (Slatkin and Rhiner, 2003).

9.3 Percutaneous vertebral cementoplasty

Instability of vertebrae due to metastatic disease can cause pain. Vertebral collapse causes pain per se, but structural change may also risk nerve root compression and precipitate spinal canal stenosis. Percutaneous vertebral cementoplasty (also known as percutaneous vertebroplasty) under radiological control, has been used to reduce pain and treat vertebral body collapse (Gangi et al., 1996) (Figure 9.2).

The analgesic mechanism of this technique is not explained solely by treating collapse, since as little as 2 ml of methylmethacrylate cement can achieve good pain relief [Gangi et al., 2003]. Indeed, stabilization of microfractures, and subsequent reduction in mechanical forces through the bone, have been postulated as analgesic mechanisms (Legroux-Gerot et al., 2004). Analgesia could also be secondary to cytotoxic and thermal destruction of tumour cells, and interference with tumour blood supply.

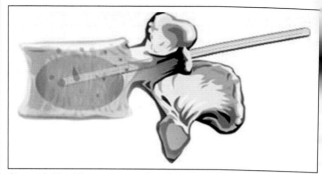

Figure 9.2 Pictorial representation of vertebroplasty at the lumbar level, showing vertebral puncture via the postero-lateral route and vertebral filling.

A study of patients with intractable pain from vertebral myeloma found that 97% patients had at least a 'moderate' reduction in pain following percutaneous vertebral cementoplasty (Cortet et al., 1997). The improvement in pain of 36/37 patients in this study was unrelated to the proportion of vertebral filling, reiterating the importance of tumour destruction rather than anatomical correction (Cotten et al., 1996).

Percutaneous vertebroplasty has been performed on patients with evidence of spinal stenosis, with or without spinal cord compression (Appel and Gilula 2004). A retrospective analysis of 23 patients found that 87% reported an improvement in pain and 22% complained of no pain at all (Appel and Gilula, 2004). Significant analgesia was maintained for up to 3 years, although concerns were raised about increased number of fractures in neighbouring vertebrae (Legroux-Gerot et al., 2004).

Cement leak is a potential problem, which can encroach upon the epidural space risking root or cord compression, and also chemothermal damage (Gangi et al., 2003). Cement embolism may also occur if there is evidence of a venous leak. However, in a case series of 868 percutaneous cementoplasty procedures for malignant and non-malignant vertebral body collapse, epidural leak was only observed in 15 cases (three had neuralgia-type pain), and asymptomatic pulmonary embolism in two cases (Gangi et al., 2003).

It should be noted that injection of methylmethacrylate is not restricted to the vertebrae, and has been reported to be successful in the management of bone pain involving the pelvic bones (Cotten et al., 1995, 1999).

Figure 9.2 is reproduced from Gangi, A., Guth, S., Imbert, J.P. et al. (2003). Percutaneous vertebioplasty: indications, technique and results. *Radio Graphics*, **23**: 10, with permission from the Radiological Society of North America (RSNA).

9.4 **Percutaneous balloon kyphoplasty**

Balloon kyphoplasty is a similar procedure to percutaneous vertebro-plasty, but involves an initial inflation of a balloon in the vertebral body, which improves vertebral alignment and generates a space to be filled with cement (Fourney et al., 2003; Gaitanis et al., 2005).

In one study of cancer and non-cancer patients with vertebral body compression fractures (of which five were secondary to osteolytic tumours), 31/32 patients experienced significant improvement in pain, in addition to achieving kyphosis correction (Gaitanis et al., 2005). In another study of cancer patients (21 with myeloma and 35 with other bony malignancies), 84% patients obtained compete relief of pain following balloon kyphoplasty (Fourney et al., 2003).

9.5 **Direct bone tumour ablation**

Another interventional strategy in bone pain management is destruc-tion of bony metastatic disease. Alcohol and phenol have been infil-trated directly into vertebral tumours under radiographic control (Gangi et al., 1996). In one study, painful osteolytic bone metastases refractory to chemo radiotherapy were treated using computed tomography (CT)-guided injections of 95% ethanol (Gangi et al., 1994). Three-quarters of the 25 patients had reduced analgesic requirements following the procedure.

Bone tumour can also be ablated by radiofrequency treatment that acts either by thermal destruction or by electromagnetic field generation (Miguel, 2000; Posteraro et al., 2004) (Figure 9.3). Goetz et al., (2004) reported 43 patients that had received radiofrequency ablation for the treatment of pain secondary to metastatic bone disease (Goetz et al., 2004): pain scores were reduced from 7.9/10 to 1.4/10 at 24 weeks post procedure, with 95% patients reporting a clinically significant reduction in pain.

Other methods of direct tumour ablation that have been used, include cryoablation, and laser ablation (Callstrom et al., 2006).

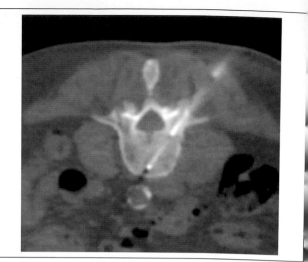

Figure 9.3 Prone CT image of radiofrequency electrode in a metastatic vertebral lesion.

References

Antila, H. and Kirvela, O. (1998). Neurolytic thoracic paravertebral block in cancer pain. A clinical report. *Acta Anaesthesiol. Scand.*, **42**, 581–5.

Appel, N.B. and Gilula, L.A. (2004). Percutaneous vertebroplasty in patients with spinal canal compromise. *Am. J. Roentgenol.*, **182**, 947–51.

Appelgren, L., Nordborg, C., Sjoberg, M., Karlsson, P.A., Nitescu, P., and Curelaru, I. (1997). Spinal epidural metastasis: implications for spinal analgesia to treat "refractory" cancer pain. *J. Pain Sympt. Management*, **13**, 25–42.

Arner, S., Lindblom, U., Meyerson, B.A., and Molander, C. (1990). Prolonged relief of neuralgia after regional anesthetic blocks. A call for further experimental and systematic clinical studies. *Pain*, **43**, 287–97.

Bedder, M.D., Burchiel, K., and Larson, A. (1991). Cost analysis of two implantable narcotic delivery systems. *J. Pain Sympt. Management*, **6**, 368–73.

Boswell, M.V., Shah, R.V., Everett, C.R. *et al.* (2005). Interventional techniques in the management of chronic spinal pain: evidence-based practice guidelines. *Pain Physn*, **8**, 1–47.

Breivik, B., Campbell, W., and Eccleston. (2002). *Clinical pain management: practical applications and procedures*. Hodder Arnold, London.

Bruera, E., and Kim, H.N. (2003). Cancer pain. *JAMA*, **290**, 2476–9.

Figure 9.3 is reproduced from Posteraro, A.F., Dupuy, D.E., and Mayo-Smith, W.W. (2004). Radiofrequency ablation of bony metastatic disease. *Clin. Radiol.*, **59**: 803–11, with permission from the Royal College of Radiologists.

Callstrom, M.R., Charboneau, J.W., Goetz, M.P. et al. (2006). Image-guided ablation of painful metastatic bone tumors: a new and effective approach to a difficult problem. *Skeletal Radiol.*, **35**, 1–15.

Candido, K., and Stevens, R.A. (2003). Intrathecal neurolytic blocks for the relief of cancer pain. *Best Pract. Res. Clin. Anaesthesiol.*, **17**, 407–28.

Coderre, T.J., Katz, J., Vaccarino, A.L., and Melzack, R. (1993). Contribution of central neuroplasticity to pathological pain: review of clinical and experimental evidence. *Pain*, **52**, 259–85.

Cortet, B., Cotton, A., Boutry, N. et al. (1997). Percutaneous vertebroplasty in patients with osteolytic metastases or multiple myeloma. *Revue du Rhumatisme* (English edn), **64**, 177–83.

Cotton, A., Deprez, X., Migaud, H., Chabanne, B., Duquesnoy, B., and Chastanet, P. (1995). Malignant acetabular osteolyses: percutaneous injection of acrylic bone cement. *Radiology*, **197**, 307–10.

Cotton, A., Dewatre, F., Cortet, B. et al. (1996). Percutaneous vertebroplasty for osteolytic metastases and myeloma: effects of the percentage of lesion filling and the leakage of methyl methacrylate at clinical follow-up. *Radiology*, **200**, 525–30.

Cotton, A., Demondion, X., Boutry, N. et al. (1999). Therapeutic percutaneous injections in the treatment of malignant acetabular osteolyses. *Radiographics*, **19**, 647–53.

Dahm, P., Nitescu, P., Appelgren, L., and Curelaru, I. (1998). Efficacy and technical complications of long-term continuous intraspinal infusions of opioid and/or bupivacaine in refractory nonmalignant pain: a comparison between the epidural and the intrathecal approach with externalized or implanted catheters and infusion pumps. *Clin. J. Pain*, **14**, 4–16.

Davis, M.P., Walsh, D., Lagman, R., and LeGrand, S.B. (2005). Controversies in pharmacotherapy of pain management. *Lancet Oncol.*, **6**, 696–704.

de Leon-Casasola, O.A. (2004). Interventional procedures for cancer pain management: when are they indicated? *Cancer Invest.*, **22**, 630–42.

Doyle, D., Hanks, G., Cherny, N.I., and Calman, K. (2004). *Oxford textbook of palliative Medicine* (3rd edn). Oxford University Press, Oxford.

Eisenach, J.C., DuPen, S., Dubois, M., Miguel, R., and Allin, D. (1995). Epidural clonidine analgesia for intractable cancer pain. The Epidural Clonidine Study Group. *Pain*, **61**, 391–9.

Erdine, S., and Talu, G.K. (1998). Cost effectiveness of implantable catheters. *Curr. Rev. Pain*, **2**, 157–62.

Fischer, H.B., Peters, T.M., Fleming, I.M., and Else, T.A. (1996). Peripheral nerve catheterization in the management of terminal cancer pain. *Regional Anesth.*, **21**, 482–5.

Fourney, D.R., Schomer, D.F., Nader, R. et al. (2003). Percutaneous vertebroplasty and kyphoplasty for painful vertebral body fractures in cancer patients. *J. Neurosurg.*, 98 (1 Suppl.), 21–30.

Gaitanis, I.N., Hadjipavlou, A.G., Katonis, P.G., Tzermiadianos, M.N., Pasku, D.S., and Patwardhan, A.G. (2005). Balloon kyphoplasty for the treatment of pathological vertebral compressive fractures. *Eur. Spine J.*, **14**, 250–60.

Gangi, A., Dietemann, J.L., Schultz, A., Mortazavi, R., Jeung, M.Y., and Roy, C. (1996). Interventional radiologic procedures with CT guidance in cancer pain management. *Radiographics*, **16**, 1289–1304.

Gangi, A., Guth, S., Imbert, J.P., Marin, H., and Dietemann, J.L. (2003). Percutaneous vertebroplasty: indications, technique, and results. *Radiographics*, **23**, e10.

Gangi, A., Kastler, B., Klinkert, A., and Dietemann, J.L. (1994). Injection of alcohol into bone metastases under CT guidance. *J. Comput. Assist. Tomogr.*, **18**, 932–5.

Goetz, M.P., Callstrom, M.R., Charboneau, J.W. *et al.* (2004). Percutaneous image-guided radiofrequency ablation of painful metastases involving bone: a multicenter study. *J. Clin. Oncol.*, **22**, 300–6.

Janson, W., and Stein, C. (2003). Peripheral opioid analgesia. *Curr. Pharmaceut. Biotechnol.*, **4**, 270–4.

Kalso, E., Heiskanen, T., Rantio, M., Rosenberg, P.H., and Vainio, A. (1996). Epidural and subcutaneous morphine in the management of cancer pain: a double-blind cross-over study. *Pain*, **67**, 443–9.

Khor, K.E., and Ditton, J.N. (1996). Femoral nerve blockade in the multidisciplinary management of intractable localized pain due to metastatic tumor: a case report. *J. Pain Sympt. Management*, **11**, 57–6.

Kim, P.S. (2005). Interventional cancer pain therapies. *Semin. Oncol.*, **32**, 194–9.

Kori, S.H., LaPerriere, J.A., Kowalski, M.B., Rodriguez, C., and Dinwoodie, W. (1997). Management of bone pain secondary to metastatic disease. *Cancer Control*, **4**, 153–7.

Lamacraft, G., and Cousins, M.J. (1997). Neural blockade in chronic and cancer pain. *Int. Anesthesiol. Clin.*, **35**, 131–53.

Lawson, A., and Siemaszko, O. (2003). Long term epidural treatment of refractory malignant and nonmalignant pain using internal and external pumps. In: Breivik, H., Campbell, W., and Eccleston, C., (ed.) *Practical applications and procedures*. Arnold, London.

Legroux-Gerot, I., Lormeau, C., Boutry, N., Cotton, A., Duquesnoy, B., and Cortet, B. (2004). Long-term follow-up of vertebral osteoporotic fractures treated by percutaneous vertebroplasty. *Clin. Rheumatol.*, **23**, 310–7.

Lordon, S.P. (2002). Interventional approach to cancer pain. *Curr. Pain Headache Rep.*, **6**, 202–6.

McMahon, S., and Koltzenburg, M. (2005). *Wall and Melzack's textbook of pain* (5th edn). Churchill Livingstone, Edinburgh.

Miguel, R. (2000). Interventional treatment of cancer pain: the fourth step in the World Health Organization analgesic ladder? *Cancer Control*, **7**, 149–56.

Nishikawa, K., Kanaya, N., Nakayama, M., Igarashi, M., Tsunoda, K., and Namiki, A. (2000). Fentanyl improves analgesia but prolongs the onset of axillary brachial plexus block by peripheral mechanism. *Anesth. Analg.*, **91**, 384–7.

Nitescu, P., Appelgren, L., and Curelaru, I. (2003). Long term intrathecal and intracisternal treatment of malignant and nonmalignant pain using external pumps. In: Breivik, H., Campbell, W., Eccleston, C. (ed.) *Practical applications and procedures*. Arnold, London.

Nitescu, P., Appelgren, L., Linder, L.E., Sjoberg, M., Hultman, E., and Curelaru, I. (1990). Epidural versus intrathecal morphine-bupivacaine: assessment of consecutive treatments in advanced cancer pain. *J. Pain Sympt. Management*, **5**, 18–26.

Peng, P., and Massicotte, E.M. (2004). Spinal cord compression from intrathecal catheter-tip inflammatory mass: case report and a review of etiology. *Regional Anesth. Pain Med.*, **29**, 237–42.

Posteraro, A.F., Dupuy, D.E., and Mayo-Smith, W.W. (2004). Radiofrequency ablation of bony metastatic disease. *Clin. Radiol.*, **59**, 803–11.

Rauck, R.L., Cherry, D., Boyer, M.F., Kosek, P., Dunn, J., and Alo, K. (2003). Long-term intrathecal opioid therapy with a patient-activated, implanted delivery system for the treatment of refractory cancer pain. *J. Pain*, **4**, 441–7.

Reale, C., Turkiewicz, A.M., and Reale, C.A. (2001). Antalgic treatment of pain associated with bone metastases. *Crit. Rev. Oncol–Hematol.*, **37**, 1–11.

Slatkin, N.E., and Rhiner, M. (2003). Phenol saddle blocks for intractable pain at end of life: report of four cases and literature review. *Am. J. Hospice Palliat. Care*, **20**, 62–6.

Smith, T.J., Coyne, P.J., Staats, P.S. *et al.* (2005). An implantable drug delivery system (IDDS) for refractory cancer pain provides sustained pain control, less drug-related toxicity, and possibly better survival compared with comprehensive medical management (CMM). *Ann. Oncol.*, **16**, 825–33.

Swerdlow, M. (1978). Intrathecal neurolysis. Anaesthesia, **33**, 733–40.

Vainio, A., and Tigerstedt, I. (1988). Opioid treatment for radiating cancer pain: oral administration vs. epidural techniques. *Acta Anaesth. Scand.*, **32**, 179–85.

World Health Organization (1996). Cancer pain relief (2nd edn). WHO, Geneva.

Yanagidate, F., and Dohi, S. (2004). Epidural oxycodone or morphine following gynaecological surgery. *Br. J. Anaesth.*, **93**, 362–7.

Chapter 10

Orthopaedic interventions

Wisam Al-Hakim, Jacob Jagiello and Timothy Briggs

10.1 Introduction

The management of patients with primary or secondary bone cancer can be extremely difficult, and requires a multidisciplinary approach that involves, amongst others, oncologists, pain specialists and orthopaedic surgeons (Anonymous, 1999). There are several indications for orthopaedic intervention, particularly refractory pain, pathological fracture, impending fracture, and associated radiculopathy or myelopathy (Harrington, 1997).

This chapter is dedicated to palliative orthopaedics, i.e. to situations where the emphasis is on treatment of symptoms, rather than on cure of the disease. The different sections have been designed to cover the treatment of pathological fractures in general, and then more specifically the treatment of malignancy involving the femur, the humerus, the pelvis and the spine. Readers are advised to consult a relevant orthopaedic textbook for further information about specific techniques.

10.2 General principles

The surgeon must take into account a number of factors when deciding if an orthopaedic intervention is justified, and also which procedure is likely to yield the best results for the patient. These include the type of tumour, the anatomical site, the overall size, the type of fracture, involvement of adjacent tissues, response to non-surgical treatment, co-morbidity and predicted prognosis. Surgery should be considered in all patients with the exception of those with a level of co-morbidity deemed too great to survive an operation.

10.2.1 Assessment

It is crucial that the correct diagnosis is made, in order to prevent inappropriate treatment being administered. It must never be assumed that a single bone lesion is metastatic in nature: if the lesion is a primary bone tumour, then the appropriate treatment is a curative resection and reconstruction with an endoprosthesis; an inappropriate fixation procedure may lead to dissemination of the tumour, which could be catastrophic for the patient. If there is any doubt regarding the tumour type, then a tissue biopsy is indicated (Tillman, 1999).

Two-view plain radiographs of the entire bone in question must be performed, since concomitant lesions can occur in the same bone, and may influence the surgical procedure performed. In addition, computed tomography and magnetic resonance imaging are very useful modalities for more accurately assessing periarticular, spinal and soft tissue involvement. Other relevant investigations must also be performed prior to surgery (e.g. routine blood tests, chest radiograph).

10.2.2 **Surgery for pathological fracture**

The aim of fixing these types of fractures is different from that of traumatic (non-pathological) fractures. Bone healing in these situations is impaired, and often the fragments do not unite together. It is therefore a priority that the operation involves a method of fracture fixation that forms a stable, strong, permanent construct, and that can allow immediate return to normal function.

Several factors have been shown to be significantly associated with rates of bone healing in these patients, including tumour type and patient survival (Gainor's criteria) (Gainor and Buchert, 1983). Specifically breast carcinoma and multiple myeloma have better rates of healing than lung or colorectal carcinoma. Importantly adjuvant treatment such as radiotherapy and chemotherapy inhibit bone healing (Wedin et al., 1999).

Fractures can be surgically managed in several different ways. The principal methods of internal fixation include application of a plate fixed across a fracture by screws, or the placement of an intramedullary rod that is secured in place by proximal and distal transverse locking screws. When these methods are contraindicated, then resection of the tumour can be followed by reconstruction using an endoprosthesis. Cement can be used in combination with the above techniques: it fills gaps left by debulking of large tumours, adds mechanical stability, and through its exothermic reaction may have a role in improving haemostasis and minimizing tumour cell contamination.

10.2.3 **Surgery for impending fracture**

Some malignant bone lesions cause symptoms in the absence of a fracture; such lesions are at risk of fracturing sometime in the future (although many do not fracture, and the symptoms settle with conservative measures). In general, metastases in long bones progress to fractures in ~25% of cases (although this rises to ~60% in the proximal femur).

Table 10.1 Mirels' scoring system for impending pathological fracture (Mirels, 1989)

Variable	Score		
	1	**2**	**3**
Site	Upper limb	Lower limb	Peritrochanteric
Pain	Mild	Moderate	Functional
Lesion	Blastic	Mixed	Lytic
Size*	<1/3	1/3 to 2/3	>2/3

*Maximum destruction of cortex in any view as seen on plain X-ray

The criteria for operating on impending fractures vary. A widely used method is Mirel's scoring system (Table 10.1) (Mirels', 1989). This uses four factors related to the likelihood of a malignant bone lesion fracturing. These include:

- the site of the lesion
- the amount of pain caused by the lesion
- whether the lesion is blastic, lytic or a combination
- the size and involvement of the lesion (defined as the maximum amount of cortex destroyed).

A score of 1–3 is given for each variable, so that the lowest total score is four and the highest total score is twelve. A score of ≤7 indicates that surgery is not needed, whereas a score of ≥9 indicates that surgery is warranted: a score of 8 means that the decision has to taken in the context of the patient and his/her disease.

Current opinion is that this scoring system is useful, but that experience is a much more accurate predictor of fracture risk. For example, patients with severe pain every time they weight-bear, in spite of appropriate analgesics and radiotherapy, are likely to benefit from surgery no matter what their calculated score.

There is mixed evidence to support the case that the outcome for surgical management of impending pathological fractures is better than that for actual fractures. Ward et al. (2003) reported a significant difference in favour of patients with impending fractures in terms of peri-operative blood loss, shorter hospital stay, greater likelihood of discharge home instead of temporary step-down facilities, and higher rates of unassisted ambulation. In contrast, Dijkstra et al., (1994) reported no significant difference in outcomes such as pain relief, physical function, complications and survival.

10.3 **Femur**

Pathological fractures are most commonly reported in the femur (~60% of all long bone involvement). The vast majority develop in the proximal femur (~80%): 50% occur in the femoral head and neck, 30% are subtrochanteric, and 20% are intertrochanteric (Sim *et al.*, 1992).

Surgery is indicated for established fractures, and in cases of lesser trochanter avulsion (pathognomonic of pathological fracture). The indications for surgery for impending fracture vary, but usually include painful lytic lesions resistant to radiotherapy, lesions of >2.5cm, cortical destruction of ≥50% (as seen on a radiograph in any view), and a Mirels score of ≥9.

The surgeon strives to reduce or eliminate pain, and return the patient to walking as soon as possible. The procedure, therefore, must provide enough stability to allow for immediate, or at least early, post-operative weight-bearing. It should be assumed that the fracture will not unite, no matter how well prepared the healing environment. Furthermore, such operations cannot be regarded as a temporary procedure, and must be designed for potentially many years of use (Jacofsky and Haidukewych, 2004).

10.3.1 **Internal fixation**

Internal fixation uses either plates and screws, or intramedullary devices.

Plates and screws

Plate fixation has been particularly used in the proximal femur, and can be effective for subtrochanteric and metaphyseal fractures. The plates act as load-bearing devices, in that they resist the forces transmitted both through and across the fracture that they are bridging.

Important factors that must be fulfilled before adopting this technique are that the joint is not involved, and that the articular surfaces are relatively intact. In addition, the surrounding bone must be strong enough to hold the screws, and so keep the construct stable (i.e. at least one cortex must be intact).

There are certain disadvantages with this technique, which have limited its use in recent years. Thus, plates are not as biomechanically strong as intramedullary rods, and more readily break over time. Furthermore, the quality of bone to which they are fixed almost inevitably worsens over time, and so the screws eventually loosen and the fixation fails. In addition, the drill holes can act as stress risers, which may lead to secondary fractures.

Intramedullary devices

Intramedullary nails fixed with proximal and distal locking screws have a number of advantages over plates. As the neutral axis of the nail and femur are similar, they act as load-sharing devices, so that forces acting on the diseased femur are supported by the metalwork as well as the native bone.

The intramedullary nails that fit into the femoral medulla are thick enough to possess a very high level of mechanical strength. They support the entire femur, which is useful if there is more than one focus of disease, or if new lesions develop over time. This type of fixation has potentially excellent long-term survival.

This technique has been improved with the use of reconstruction-type nails that place interlocking proximal screws through the head and neck of the femur, which increases the resistance to angular and rotational stresses and protects against fracture in the regions most frequently affected.

However, there are limitations to the use of intramedullary nails. For example, if there is extensive destruction of bone, or involvement of the femoral head/neck or hip joint, then sometimes patients are treated more appropriately by resection and reconstruction with an endoprosthesis (see below). Similarly, densely sclerotic lesions, or metaphyseal fragments that cannot be adequately stabilized, will require alternative forms of surgery.

10.3.2 **Endoprostheses**

The other principal method used is bone tumour resection and reconstruction with an endoprosthesis (Keating *et al.,* 1990). These techniques are generally reserved for large, or periarticular, lesions.

A hemiarthroplasty can be used to replace the head and neck of a diseased femur. For concomitant distal lesions, long-stem implants can be used to provide additional support. If there is suspected involvement of the acetabulum, then depending on the extent of involvement, a total hip replacement can be used. However, most studies advocate the use of hemiarthroplasty alone (when possible), as this has fewer distressing complications such as dislocation of the hip.

Massive endoprostheses can be used if there is a great deal of bone destruction, or if the tumour is likely to be insensitive to post-operative radiation or chemotherapy. They can replace the proximal, distal, midshaft and even the whole of the femur (Figures 10.1 and 10.2). Not surprisingly, these are the most extensive and technically demanding procedures. The functional outcome depends upon the extent of the disease, and the amount of soft tissue resected around the hip joint. Instability, dislocation, infection and deep vein thrombosis are all significant complications.

Figure 10.1 (a) Massive endoprosthesis for replacing proximal femur (b) Endoprosthesis *in situ*

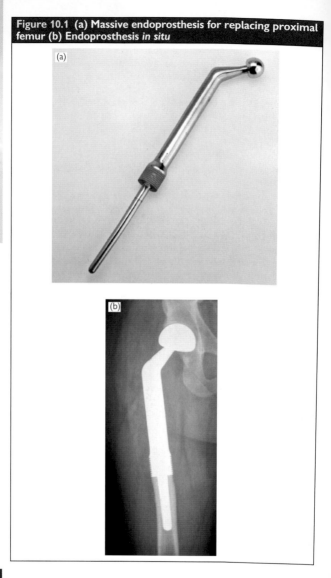

Figure 10.2 (a) Massive endoprosthesis for replacing distal femur. (b) Endoprosthesis *in situ*

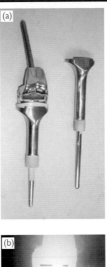

(a)

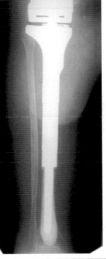

(b)

10.3.4 **Other options**
Other options are available to patients who do not qualify for the above. Large infected tumours, or those with cutaneus ulceration, or those with neurovascular involvement may require amputation. This can reduce pain and, with the aid of a suitable prosthesis, can also improve function.

Cast immobilization can be used for patients with extensive local disease, and also in terminally ill patients.

10.4 **Humerus**

This is the second most commonly affected long bone. The majority of fractures occur in the middle third of the humerus, followed by the proximal third, and then the distal third.

There have been fewer studies that have looked into humeral surgery. However, the indications for surgery are similar to what has been previously mentioned, although the principles of surgery are somewhat different (Dijkstra et al., 1996). Proximal humeral lesions often involve the rotator cuff musculature, or adjacent tuberosities, meaning that full restoration of function is unlikely, and so not as great a focus in the mind of the operating surgeon.

10.4.1 **Internal fixation**
Internal fixation using plates has been used to good effect in this situation. The stresses exerted are low in comparison to the femur, and so the likelihood of fatigue fracture is reduced. However, there is a risk of soft tissue injury, which can lead to problematic nerve palsies (e.g. wrist drop).

The intramedullary canal of a humerus is smaller than that of a femur, particularly in female or small patients. This means that only thin devices can be accommodated, and thus truly rigid fixation can be difficult to achieve. Rush pins are thin intramedullary devices that can be used to fix fractures, and several of them can be used simultaneously to provide increased rigidity and support.

10.4.2 **Endoprostheses**
Again, lesions that are not amenable to these fixation techniques will sometimes require resection and replacement with an endoprosthesis (Figure 10.3).

10.5 **Pelvis**

The indications for pelvic surgery follow the same pattern as for malignant bone disease elsewhere, i.e. pain that responds poorly to conservative measures (e.g. opioid analgesics, radiotherapy), and pelvic fractures causing pain and/or compromising function.

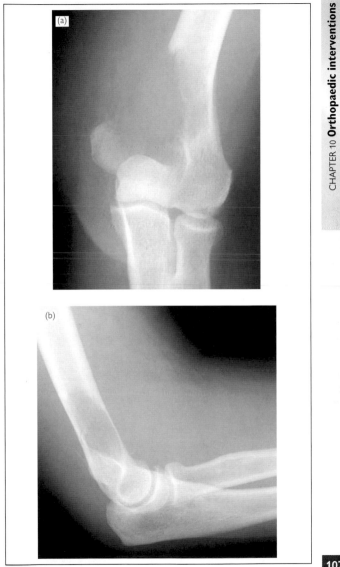

Figure 10.3 (a) Anteroposterior view of osteolytic lesion in distal humerus.
(b) Lateral view of same osteolytic lesion in distal humerus.

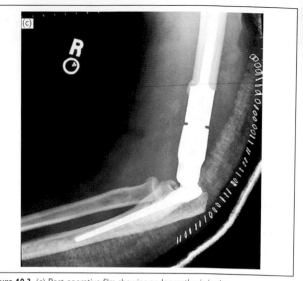

Figure 10.3 (c) Post-operative film showing endoprosthesis *in situ*.

Tumours affecting the ischium or ilium can sometimes be excised without the need for extensive reconstruction. However, peri-acetabular lesions will need an operation that not only excises the tumour, but also employs a reconstructive technique that restores force transmission along anatomical axes.

The principles of all periacetabular operations are to resect the tumour adequately, preserve as much intact bone as possible, obtain haemostasis (as pelvic surgery inevitably produces significant blood loss), and restore a mechanically sound support for ambulation. There are two methods of reconstruction, which are most widely practised:

1. Reconstruction using stabilising pins and cement, with or without a prosthetic acetabular component (Figure 10.4)—this technique is used for smaller tumours.
2. Reconstruction using a hemipelvic autograft, allograft, or endoprosthesis—this technique is used for larger tumours.

In the first technique the resection defect can be reinforced, and a lattice created, with the use of stabilizing pins. The first set of pins is inserted in a retrograde manner through the surgical defect and anchored into the medial iliac crest or sacro-iliac joint; the second set is inserted in an anterograde manner from the lateral iliac crest

Figure 10.4 (a) A typical Stanmore acetabular prosthesis with an implant for replacement of the femoral head and neck. **(b)** Acetabular prosthesis *in situ*

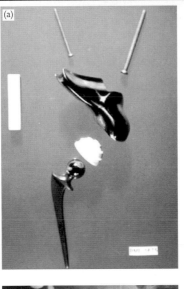

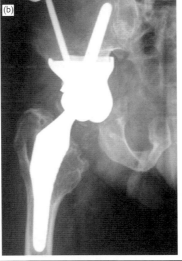

to the surgical defect. This creates a bed upon which a cemented acetabular, or similar pelvic prosthesis, can achieve good fixation.

In the second technique, a custom-built endoprosthesis can be used, although reports suggest that they have a significant failure rate, mainly because the fixation to the remaining bone is liable to loosen. Other studies have shown that autoclaved autograft can be used in combination with pins and cement (Harrington, 1992). Thus, after the hemipelvis has been excised, and all tumour has been stripped away, there is sometimes enough intact acetabular surface to form an adequate joint, and sufficient remaining bone to form an intact pelvic ring. In such instances the specimen undergoes autoclaving (and even irradiation if a high grade cancer is involved), and is then reinserted into the remaining pelvis. Allografts using vascularized fibula have also been used in this situation.

Other techniques have been employed to manage periarticular disease, but these are associated with poor functional outcomes, e.g. iliofemoral arthrodesis (fusion of femur to ilium), ischiofemoral arthrodesis (fusion of femur to ischium), use of so-called 'saddle' prostheses.

Overall functional outcomes are generally very promising, with improvements shown in the vast majority of studies (Marco et al., 2000; Satcher et al., 2003). The length of stay and rehabilitation process is shortest in those who undergo reconstruction with pins and cement. Outcomes have also been described as being better in patients with primary bone tumours than in those with metastatic bone disease.

As expected, there are complications associated with these operations (Abudu et al., 1997). Haematoma and visceral injury are early/intermediate post-operative complications. Wound dehiscence is widely reported, which is generally due to infection or local progression of the tumour. Deep vein thrombosis is also widely reported. Furthermore, dislocation and late fixation failure are reported as commonly as 6–21% in case series (Satcher et al., 2003).

Orthopaedic intervention is justified in many of those patients who can tolerate such a procedure, with the benefits generally outweighing the risks (Healey and Brown, 2000). However, due to the challenging nature of these operations, they are best undertaken in specialized tertiary centres.

10.6 Spine

The spine is noted to be the most common site for skeletal metastases. The thoracic spine is the most common site of disease (70%), followed by the lumbar spine (20%), and the cervical spine (10%) (Byrne, 1992; Gerszten et al., 2000; Gilbert et al., 1978). Metastatic spinal disease can arise from three locations: the vertebral column (85%), the paravertebral region (10–15%), and rarely the epidural or subarachnoid space (<5%) (Byrne, 1992; Gerszten et al., 2000; Gilbert et al., 1978). Moreover, 14% of patients have involvement of a single vertebral body, and the remaining 86% have multiple vertebral bodies affected (O'Donoghue et al., 1997).

The indications for spinal surgery are intractable pain unresponsive to non operative measures, the presence of spinal instability, and/or the presence of neurological deficit (i.e. nerve root compression, spinal cord compression).

The orthopaedic principles underlying management are debulking of tumour mass, decompression of neural structures, stabilization to allow weight-bearing, and realignment of spinal deformity. Furthermore, the surgical goals should include the provision of fixation to last the lifetime of the patient.

Management is influenced by a number of different factors, including the topography of the problem and, particularly, the prognosis of the patient. Several surgical evaluation systems have been developed, including the so-called Tokuhashi scoring system (Tokuhashi et al., 1990), which enables the surgeon to minimize the surgical intervention in patients with an estimated survival of <3 months.

In the palliative setting, isolated posterior stabilization gives satisfactory attenuation of pain. There is a variety of posterior stabilization techniques in use for patients with spinal tumours (e.g. pedicle screws, Harrington distraction rods) (Galasko et al., 2000; Fourney et al., 2001). In other instances, an anterior or combined approach involving tumour resection as well as appropriate spinal stabilization is utilized (Figure 10.5) (Harrington, 1984; Galasko et al., 2000). (These techniques are more invasive in nature, and so associated with a greater risk of significant morbidity.)

Surgical treatment of spinal metastases by means of decompression together with spinal stabilization has proved beneficial in providing substantial improvement in the functional status of >80% patients (Onimus et al., 1996). Thus, patients with pain achieved improved analgesia, whilst patients with neurological deficits achieved improved neurological function. Indeed, 70% patients that were unable to walk before surgery (due to pain and/or neurological deficit), were able to walk following surgery and rehabilitation.

In another study by Patchell et al., (2005) patients with spinal cord compression treated with surgery and radiotherapy retained the ability to walk significantly longer than those treated with radiotherapy alone. Thus, surgery permitted most patients to remain ambulatory and continent for the remainder of their lives, while patients treated with radiation alone spent approximately two-thirds of their remaining time unable to walk and being incontinent.

Figure 10.5 Lateral view of a posterior stabilization construct

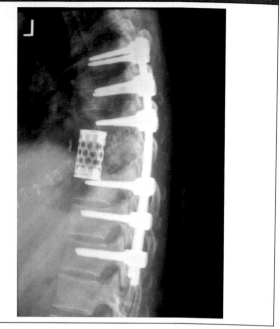

References

Abudu, A., Grimer, R.J., Cannon, S.R., Carter, S.R., and Sneath, R.S. (1997). Reconstruction of the hemipelvis after the excision of malignant tumours. Complications and functional outcome. *J. Bone Joint Surg. (Br. Vol.)*, **79-B**, 773–9.

Anonymous, (1999). British Association of Surgical Oncology Guidelines. The management of metastatic bone disease in the United Kingdom. The Breast Specialty Group of the British Association of Surgical Oncology. *Eur. J. Surg. Oncol.*, **25**, 3–23.

Byrne, T.N. (1992). Spinal cord compression from epidural metastases. *New England J. Med.*, **327**, 614–9.

Dijkstra, S., Wiggers, T., van Geel, B.N., and Boxma, H. (1994). Impending and actual pathological fractures in patients with bone metastases of the long bones. A retrospective study of 233 surgically treated fractures. *Eur. J. Surg.*, **160**, 535–42.

Dijkstra, S., Stapert, J., Boxma, H., and Wiggers, T. (1996). Treatment of pathological fractures of the humeral shaft due to bone metastases: a comparison of intramedullary locking nail and plate osteosynthesis with adjunctive bone cement. *Eur. J. Surg. Oncol.*, **22**, 621–6.

Fourney, D.R., Abi-Said, D., Lang, F.F., McCutcheon, I.E., and Gokaslan, Z.L. (2001). Use of pedicle screw fixation in the management of malignant spinal disease: experience in 100 consecutive procedures. *J. Neurosurg.*, **94** (1 Suppl.), 25–37.

Galasko, C.S., Norris, H.E., and Crank, S. (2000). Spinal instability secondary to metastatic cancer. *J. Bone Joint Surg.* (Amer. Vol.), **82**, 570–6.

Gainor, B.J., and Buchert, P. (1983). Fracture healing in metastatic bone disease. *Clin. Orthop. Related Res.*, **178**, 297–302.

Gerszten, P.C., and Welch WC (2000). Current surgical management of metastatic spinal disease. Oncology (Huntington), **14**, 1013–24.

Gilbert, R.W., Kim, J.H., and Posner, J.B. (1978). Epidural spinal cord compression from metastatic tumor: diagnosis and treatment. *Ann. Neurol.*, **3**, 40–51.

Harrington, K.D. (1984). Anterior cord decompression and spinal stabilization for patients with metastatic lesions of the spine. *J. Neurosurg.*, **61**, 107–17.

Harrington, K.D. (1992). The use of pelvic allografts or autoclaved grafts for reconstruction after wide resections of malignant tumors of the pelvis. *J. Bone Joint Surg. Amer. Vol.*, **74**, 331–41.

Harrington, K.D. (1997). Orthopedic surgical management of skeletal complications of malignancy. *Cancer*, **80** (8 Suppl.), 1614–27.

Healey, J.H., and Brown, H.K. (2000). Complications of bone metastases: surgical management. *Cancer*, **88** (12 Suppl.), 2940–51.

Jacofsky, D.J., and Haidukewych, G.J. (2004). Management of pathological fractures of the proximal femur: state of the art. *J. Orthop. Trauma*, **18**, 459–69.

Keating, J.F., Burke, T., and Macauley, P. (1990). Proximal femoral replacement for pathological fracture. *Injury*, **21**, 231–3.

Marco, R.A., Sheth, D.S., Boland, P.J., Wunder, J.S., Siegel, J.A., and Healey, J.H. (2000). Functional and oncological outcome of acetabular reconstruction for the treatment of metastatic disease. *J. Bone Joint Surg. (Amer. Vol.)*, **82-A**, 642–51.

Mirels, H. (1989). Metastatic disease in long bones. A proposed scoring system for diagnosing impending pathological fractures. *Clin. Orthop. Related Res.*, **249**, 256–64.

O'Donoghue, D.S., Howell, A., Bundred, N.J., and Walls, J. (1997). Orthopaedic management of structurally significant bone destruction in breast cancer metastases. *J. Bone Joint Surg. (Br. Vol.)*, **79-B** (Suppl. 1), 98.

Onimus, M., Papin, P., and Gangolff, S. (1996). Results of surgical treatment of spinal thoracic and lumbar metastases. *Eur. Spine J.*, **5**, 407–11.

Patchell, R.A., Tibbs, P.A., Regine, W.F. *et al.* (2005). Direct decompressive surgical resection in the treatment of spinal cord compression caused by metastatic cancer: a randomised trial. *Lancet*, **366**, 643–8.

Satcher Jr, R.L., O'Donnell, R.J., and Johnston, J.O. (2003). Reconstruction of the pelvis after resection of tumors about the acetabulum. *Clin. Orthop. Related Res.*, **409**, 209–17.

Sim, F.H. (1992). Metastatic bone disease of the pelvis and femur. *Instruct. Course Lect.*, **41**, 317–27.

Tillman, R.M. (1999). The role of the Orthopaedic Surgeon in metastatic disease of the appendicular skeleton. *J. Bone Joint Surg. (Br. Vol.)*, **81-B**, 1–2.

Tokuhashi, Y., Matsuzaki, H., Toriyama, S., Kawano, H., and Ohsaka, S. (1990). Scoring system for the preoperative evaluation of metastatic spine tumor prognosis. *Spine*, **15**, 1110–3.

Ward, W.G., Holsenbeck, S., Dorey, F.J., Spang, J., and Howe, D. (2003). Metastatic disease of the femur: surgical treatment. *Clin. Orthop. Related Res.*, **415** (Suppl.), S230–44.

Wedin, R., Bauer, H.C., and Wersall, P. (1999). Failures after operation for skeletal metastatic lesions of long bones. *Clin. Orthop. Related Res.*, **358**, 128–39.

Index